W9-CSN-518

Global Kitchen

A Cookbook of
Vegetarian Favorites from
The Expanding Light Yoga Retreat

Diksha McCord

crystal clarity **publishers**
nevada city, california

Crystal Clarity Publishers, Nevada City, CA 95959
Copyright © 2002, 1999, 1997 Blanche Agassy McCord
All rights reserved. Published 2012.

First edition 1997. Second edition 1999.
Third edition 2002. Fourth edition 2012.

Printed in China.
ISBN13: 978-1-56589-102-9
ePub ISBN: 978-1-56589-504-1

Previously published under the title of: The Expanding Light Cookbook
ISBN: 1-56589-128-7

Cover and book design by Crystal Clarity Publishers
Illustrations for the chapter title pages and appendices by Kaleigh Surber
Additional illustrations by C. A. Starner Schuppe
and Dover Publications *Food and Drink Illustrations* by Susan Gaber

www.crystalclarity.com
800.424.1055 or 530.478.7600
clarity@crystalclarity.com

Preface to the Third Edition

We're delighted to offer you this revised edition of *Global Kitchen*. Previously *The Expanding Light Cookbook*, we have changed the title to reflect the international nature of the recipes.

As before, every recipe is simple, easy to use, and delicious. You'll find terrific vegetable, grain and bean dishes, soups, salad dressings, and quick breads. Many of these recipes are from Indian, Middle Eastern, Japanese, Thai, Italian, and Mexican cuisines. A few of the recipes use dairy, but as before, the vast majority are non-dairy.

By popular request, we've added a wide selection of suggested menus for lunches and dinners during the various seasons of the year, plus an index of recipes by region.

We hope you'll enjoy this new book.

Diksha McCord

Contents

Acknowledgments

It is my joy to present these recipes from *The Expanding Light* retreat. For the past 6 years I have been gathering, testing, and refining these recipes, as well as inventing a few of my own. I offer my deepest gratitude to Ananda's many wonderful cooks, who have inspired me and contributed their recipes to this cookbook. Particularly helpful were Viki Scatchard, Jillian Popkie, Graziella Arnoldi, Sadhana Devi Helin, Jyoti Spearin, Benjamin Bronston, Julie Howard, and Elizabeth Hughes.

Special thanks also to: Mary Oesterle and many others for their help in testing the recipes; Kaleigh Surber and Christine Starner Schuppe for their fine artwork; Emily Finegold and Cheryl Savan for typing the recipes into the computer; to Peter Schuppe for helping edit, assemble, and typeset this edition; to all the guests and staff at *The Expanding Light* for their encouragement and feedback; and to my husband Gyandev (Rich) McCord for his support and vision, and for turning the original collection of recipes into an actual book.

Finally, I wish to thank Swami Kriyananda (J. Donald Walters) for creating *Ananda* and *The Expanding Light*, and for inspiring me—and many, many others—to reach for the very highest in life. In appreciation, we have begun each section of recipes in this book with a quotation from one of his books, *Secrets of Radiant Health and Well-Being*.

I hope you enjoy these recipes. I think you will be amazed at how easy it is to create a delicious meal that is also easy to digest, leaving you feeling light and energetic. Please let me know how the recipes turn out for you!

Yours in joyful and healthful cooking,

Diksha McCord

Introduction

Tested recipes from thirty years of serving guests with loving hearts and hands.

An interview with the author, Diskha McCord:

Where did you learn to cook for a spiritual retreat?

Diksha: I've lived throughout the world and absorbed many vegetarian traditions—including macrobiotic, Ayurvedic, and Mexican. While I was growing up in Israel, I learned Kosher vegetarian cooking. When I was living and studying in Kyoto, Japan, I learned Temple Cooking from Buddhist monks. Through my studies of Hindu and yogic traditions, I learned Ayurvedic cooking theories and techniques. The cooking I have learned has always had spiritual undertones.

What is the secret to good vegetarian cooking?

Diksha: The secret is learning how to make vegetarian food that appeals to everyone. We've been serving guests vegetarian cuisine since *The Expanding Light* retreat opened in 1968. Thousands of guests have helped us test our recipes. We're offering this cookbook because guests have long urged us to offer them a way to prepare this same wonderful food at home, and now we can pass these secrets on to you.

What's unique about these recipes?

Diksha: These recipes are tested, tested, tested. The cooking procedures are simple, and the ingredients are available in most local markets—this is a big plus. Most people want wonderful meals without having to hunt all over town for exotic ingredients. We're offering 140 nutritious recipes—only three with dairy, and two with eggs. These recipes also reflect one of our basic philosophies at *The Expanding Light*: we strive to bring out the unique, natural flavors of food in creative ways using subtle spicing and carefully selected cooking techniques.

We keep individual dishes simple to make—you don't have to be Julia Child! Then, we combine these individual dishes so that there's a variety of flavors, colors, and textures in each meal. We've also offered menu ideas so you can create a feast for the eyes as well as for the taste buds.

How did you test your recipes?

Diksha: Over the years thousands of guests have tried these recipes and commented on them. Only the recipes they *really* liked made it into the book. Throughout the time I was working on the cookbook, I'd always prepare a small portion for those guests who wanted a sample to taste. Americans are very polite—if they don't like something they don't say anything. When guests don't like something, they're quiet and keep silent. By really listening to the guests I began to learn what they'd like. I'd ask for comments and find ways to improve my recipes from suggestions I'd get from the guests.

What is unique about cooking for guests at a yoga retreat?

Diksha: We need to be able to prepare light food that keeps the guests energetic so they're able to do yoga and meditation. The food can't be too stimulating—it needs to also keep the guests calm and centered. The challenge in cooking for yoga and meditation students is how to bring out the natural flavors of vegetables and grains, yet keep the tastes exciting and not dull. We avoid junk foods, but we work hard to find the foods that will satisfy guests so they don't have junk food cravings.

What have you learned from cooking at your retreat that leads to healthier lives?

Diksha: There is much more to a healthy diet than just eating food that you know is healthy for you. It's good to eat in a harmonious environment. Often the guests eat meals here in silence, so they eat consciously, not hastily, which is better for your digestion. Through the types of foods we use and the techniques we use to prepare the food, people feel nourished and satisfied on a much deeper level.

Guests tell me they have fewer cravings for junk foods when they're eating at the retreat. They also tell me they feel more grounded and don't require stimulants like coffee and chocolate. Many doctors are proclaiming that a vegetarian diet is better for the body and the heart and one's health in general. The recipes in my book are low-fat, yet very satisfying. The result is that the food is wholesome, simple and tasty; it's not bland. It's delicious food that's good for you.

The food at The Expanding Light has received rave reviews—even by meat-eaters! How do you satisfy them?

Diksha: For meat-eaters I make sure to have heavier dishes that are also healthier. If you're a meat eater and then switch to eating vegetarian foods, these heavier foods can be more satisfying. I fix things like Mexican Rice Casserole or Pad Thai with tofu, vegetables and peanuts. Our Spinach Tofu Pie tastes just like Greek Spanakopitta—people can't tell that there's no cheese in it. Our Mexican food recipes are very popular with first-time vegetarians.

How do you handle the need to have protein in the diet?

Diksha: By using different beans with different spices and herbs that aid one's digestion. For instance, I use tofu, grains, nuts and seeds, which are high in protein. Tahini, which is made from sesame seeds, makes an ideal and tasty base for vegetarian sauces. Several of my recipes include quinoa, which is a grain that is actually a complete protein.

What do you do for those who crave sweets?

Diksha: Instead of sweets, I added a whole section of breads—yeasted and non-yeasted. These breads are easy to make, wholesome, and they replace the need for heavy sweet desserts. For instance, the *Zucchini Dessert Bread*, which has a cake texture, is very popular. Our *Spinach Stuffed Bread*, *Garlic Potato Bread*, and *Rosemary Olive Bread* are all very popular and we make them fresh daily at the retreat. These are nurturing foods that satisfy the hunger for sweets.

What recipes do guests say they love the most?

Diksha: People really like the *Maple Sesame Tofu* because it's a combination of sweet and salty tastes. The *Kale Sunflower Salad*, which may sound strange, is a big hit as well. I make it with a marinade that makes it very tasty. *Millet Patties* with our *Mushroom Gravy* as well as the *Sweet Zucchini Salad* are very popular, as are our *Lemon Ginger Dressing* and *Vitality Dressing*. We plan menus ahead for a whole week, making sure that there are balanced meals and a variety for our guests, who often stay here for a week or a month.

What do you do at The Expanding Light to make the food taste better?

Diksha: During the entire cooking process it's very important to have a positive and loving attitude—so we consciously do things that will help the cooks become more calm and centered. We always offer a simple prayer before cooking, and I never cook when I'm angry or upset, as these vibrations will go into the food and the guests will feel it. We treat the food with respect, love and focused attention.

The way we handle it, the way we wash it—the whole process is done with care. We play only soft and calming music during preparation and cooking. I have a little altar in the kitchen with some flowers and maybe a candle burning to keep the mood sacred. I allow Spirit to flow through me, through my hands and heart and into the food I'm preparing.

Together with the guests, we bless the food before we eat as an act of appreciation and gratitude. We sing the prayer all together, so the entire meal becomes an uplifting experience. I began to discover that when I used this process, guests would unanimously enjoy the food much more—to the extent that they would seek me out and personally come into the kitchen and thank me for the meals.

As you explore these recipes, keep in mind that the most important ingredient for successful cooking is your own "vibration." If you cook with focused attention, joy, kindness and love, this will be reflected in the appearance and taste of the food—and in the compliments you receive.

How to Use This Book

Preparation and Baking Times

The preparation time shown for each recipe refers to preliminary tasks such as chopping, sautéing, blending, stirring, etc. If other tasks are required—e.g., baking or marinating—their times are listed separately. Of course, preparation times will vary from person to person, depending on experience. Even baking times can vary, depending on the quantities you're baking or the altitude at which you live.

Suggested Seasons for These Recipes

Your choice of a menu for a meal depends on many factors, not the least of which is the season of the year. In part, this is because of the seasonal nature of most vegetables. More important, however, is the fact that foods have subtle warming or cooling effects on the body—regardless of the serving temperature of the food.

For example, zucchini has a cooling effect, and therefore it's best to serve it in warmer weather; butternut squash has a warming effect, and therefore it's best in cooler weather. However, spicing and cooking techniques can alter these effects, making, for example, some zucchini dishes also appropriate for cooler weather.

To help you plan meals with these effects in mind, each recipe in this book suggests the seasons during which it will be most suitable.

Multiplying Recipes

As with all recipes, some ingredients in these recipes should not be scaled up proportionately when cooking for a larger number of people than indicated. This is especially true for spices and oils; scaling up the amounts will usually over-spice the food or make it too oily.

You'll want to experiment to find out how to adjust a particular recipe for larger quantities. It's best to keep a light hand while you're experimenting—it's easier to add more than it is to take some out!

Use of Oils

Some of these recipes call for sautéing ingredients in ghee or oil. Please keep in mind that, for a healthier—if slightly plainer-tasting—version, you can sauté in water instead.

If you want less fat than an oil sauté, but more flavor than a water sauté, you can begin with a water sauté, then drizzle in a very small amount of oil or melted ghee when the sautéing is complete.

Special Preparation and Cooking Procedures

Some recipes in this book require certain general procedures not described within the recipes themselves. You'll find those procedures in the following places:

How to:	Page reference:
Cook beans	86
Cook grains	106
Roast grains, nuts & seeds	106
Cut vegetables into shapes	Appendix A, 182
Shape breads and rolls	Appendix B, 183
Make ghee	Appendix C, 184
Make patties	Appendix D, 195

Glossary

Almost all of the ingredients specified in this cookbook will be familiar to you. However, a few are less common; these are described in Appendix E (page 186).

Soups

The Secret of Radiant Health and Well-Being is ...

To become conscious of colors as channels of energy. Choose foods for their diversity of colors. Color diversity will help ensure that your diet has the proper balance.

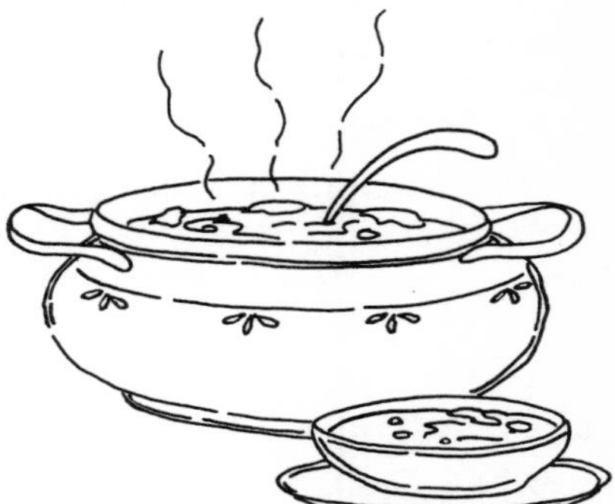

Cauliflower Soup

An outstanding soup that people ask for again and again.

Preparation time: 10 minutes
Cooking time: 20 minutes

Serves: 6
All Year

Sauté lightly:

1/3 cup olive oil
1 onion, sliced
1 carrot, peeled and cut into thin rounds
2 stalks celery, chopped
1 russet potato, peeled and cut into chunks

Add:

4 cups water
1 head cauliflower, chopped

Bring to a boil and simmer for about 20 minutes or until vegetables are soft. Allow to cool for 10 minutes. Purée in a food processor or with hand blender. Transfer to serving container and stir in:

1 tablespoon salt (or to taste)
1 teaspoon paprika
1/4 cup fresh parsley, minced, or
1 1/2 tablespoons dried parsley
1 pinch cayenne (optional)

Garnish with parsley sprig and dash of paprika.

Serving idea: Serve with Basic Whole Wheat Bread or Whole Wheat Biscuits.

Variation:

Substitute broccoli for cauliflower.

Potato Mushroom Soup

A hearty, healthy, non-dairy variation of cream of mushroom soup.

Preparation time: 20 minutes
Cooking time: 20 – 25 minutes
Serves: 8 – 10
All Year

Bring to a boil and simmer until potatoes are soft:

8 cups water
6 russet potatoes, peeled and cut into 1" cubes

Strain and return water to pot. Set potatoes aside.

While potatoes are cooking, sauté until onions are golden brown:

3 tablespoons sunflower oil
3 cups onions, sliced

Blend potatoes and onions together in a food processor or with hand blender. Once blended, return mixture to soup pot. Stir so that the water and potato-onion mixture is combined.

Sauté for 5 minutes:

2 – 4 tablespoons olive oil
12 mushrooms, cut into quarters

Add the sautéed mushrooms into the blended soup and combine with:

¼ cup tamari or Bragg Liquid Aminos (or to taste)
2 teaspoons salt (or to taste)
½ teaspoon black pepper

Serving idea: Serve with minced fresh parsley and sour cream on the side.

Variation:

Blend only half the amount of potatoes and onions in a food processor for coarser texture and add ½ tablespoon Herbs De Provence.

Barley Vegetable Soup

A rich soup with a satisfying texture.

Preparation time: 15 minutes
Cooking time: 30 minutes

Serves: 6 – 8
Spring, Autumn

Bring to a boil and simmer until all water is absorbed:

4½ cups water
1½ cups barley
½ teaspoon salt

Meanwhile, sauté for 5 minutes:

3 tablespoons sunflower oil
1 potato, peeled and cut into chunks
1 medium carrot, peeled and cut into chunks
1 stalk celery, chopped
½ medium onion, cut into chunks

Add:

4 cups water

Bring to a boil and simmer for 20 minutes. Allow to cool for 10 minutes. Then blend all vegetables together in a food processor—this creates the broth for the soup. Set aside.

Sauté for 5 minutes:

3 tablespoons olive oil
½ medium onion, minced
1 stalk celery, minced
2 small zucchini, cut into half rounds
1 cup broccoli florets, cut into small pieces
1 medium carrot, peeled and cut into rounds
1 cup cauliflower florets, cut into small pieces

Mix in a pot the vegetable broth, cooked barley, and sautéed vegetables. Cook for another 10 minutes together. Add more water if needed and add salt (2 teaspoons, or to taste).

Barley Root Vegetable Soup

A rich, hearty soup with a satisfying texture.

Preparation time: 30 minutes Serves: 8
Cooking time: 60 minutes Autumn, Winter

In a small pot bring to a boil and simmer until all water is absorbed:

3 cups water
1 cup barley

In another pot sauté for 5 minutes or until golden:

1 medium onion, minced

Add and sauté for about 5 minutes:

2 celery stalks, minced
1 large carrot or parsnip, peeled and cut into quarter rounds
1 cup yams, peeled and cubed
2 cups green cabbage, minced
2 cups mushrooms, sliced

Sprinkle, then stir in:

4 tablespoons garbanzo flour or unbleached white flour

Add and bring to a boil:

8 cups water

Add:

4 tablespoons powdered vegetable broth
cooked barley

Simmer until vegetables and barley are soft. Then add:

¼ cup fresh parsley, minced
¼ cup fresh dill, minced (or 1 teaspoon dried dill weed)
1 tablespoon salt (or to taste)
½ teaspoon black pepper

Split Pea Soup

Delicious and satisfying, especially for a cool-weather meal.

Preparation time: 20 minutes
Cooking time: 60 – 75 minutes

Serves: 4
Spring, Autumn, Winter

Place in a large soup pot:

1 cup dry split peas
4 cups water
2 bay leaves
1 teaspoon salt

Bring to a boil, cover, and simmer for 45 – 60 minutes. (Stir often to keep split peas from burning or sticking to bottom of pot. A flame diffuser is helpful, too.) When split peas get soft, discard bay leaves.

Meanwhile, sauté until onions are translucent:

3 tablespoons sunflower oil
1 small onion, minced
3 cloves of garlic, peeled and minced

Add:

1 medium carrot, peeled and cut into half rounds
1 cup mushrooms, sliced

Sauté for an additional 5 minutes. Add sautéed vegetables to split peas and simmer together for 15 minutes.

Add:

2 tablespoons tamari or Bragg Liquid Aminos
¼ teaspoon black pepper
salt to taste

Before serving, mix in:

1 tablespoon sesame seeds, roasted
2 – 4 tablespoons fresh parsley, minced

Serving idea: Excellent with Plain Rice, Basic Whole Wheat Bread or Whole Wheat Biscuits, and Potato-Garlic Spread.

Spinach Yam Soup

Delightfully different—sweet and very tasty. Great for a cold day.

Preparation time: 30 minutes
Cooking time: 20 minutes

Serves: 4
Autumn, Winter

Put in a pot:

3 cups water
4 cups yams, peeled and cut into cubes
1 large carrot, peeled and cut into rounds
2 stalks celery, cut into diagonals

Bring to a boil, then simmer for 20 minutes.

Meanwhile, sauté in a separate pan for 5–8 minutes:

2–4 tablespoons olive oil
4 cloves garlic, peeled and whole
8 ounces frozen, chopped spinach (thawed and drained)

When yams, carrots and celery are soft, let cool for 10 minutes. Then purée in a blender, food processor or with hand blender. Return to pot and stir in:

¼ teaspoon powdered ginger
¼ teaspoon black pepper
1 tablespoon tamari or Bragg Liquid Aminos
1 tablespoon fresh lemon juice

Discard garlic from sautéed spinach. Add spinach to puréed soup.

Serving idea: Serve with Basic Whole Wheat Bread.

Butternut Coconut Soup

A rich and elegant soup with a velvet texture. Great for a festive meal.

Preparation time: 20 minutes
Cooking time: 50 – 60 minutes

Serves: 4
Spring, Autumn, Winter

In a large pot, sauté until golden:

2 tablespoons butter or ghee
1 medium onion, minced
3 cloves garlic, peeled and minced

Add:

6 cups butternut squash, peeled and cubed
2 cups vegetable broth (2 cups boiling water plus 1 tablespoon vegetable broth powder) or vegetable stock

Bring to boil. Reduce heat, cover and simmer until butternut squash are soft, approximately 30 minutes. Add ½ cup to 1 cup water if needed. Add:

2 teaspoons maple syrup (optional)
½ teaspoon allspice
⅛ teaspoon dried crushed red chile pepper

Purée soup in blender or with hand blender until smooth. Return soup to pot. Bring to simmer. Add:

1½ cups canned unsweetened coconut milk

Simmer 5 – 10 minutes. Add:

½ teaspoon salt (or to taste)
¼ teaspoon black pepper

For elegant presentation, ladle soup into individual bowls and sprinkle with unsweetened coconut flakes and cilantro leaves.

Serving idea: Serve with Whole Wheat Biscuits and Sunflower Kale Salad or with Lemon Rice and Maple Sesame Tofu.

Squash Soup

Bright, light, sweet, and delicious.

Preparation time: 30 minutes
Cooking time: 25 minutes
Serves: 6
Autumn, Winter

Sauté in a pot until onions are golden:

2 tablespoons sesame oil
2 tablespoons olive oil
2 cups onions, minced
2 tablespoons fresh ginger, peeled and grated

Add:

8 cups butternut squash, peeled, seeded and cubed
4 cups water

Bring to a boil and add:

2 tablespoons powdered vegetable broth

Simmer for 20 minutes or until squash is soft. Cool for 10 minutes and purée in a blender or food processor until smooth.

Stir in:

2½ tablespoons fresh lemon juice
1 teaspoon ground coriander
1 teaspoon nutmeg
½ teaspoon ground cinnamon
½ teaspoon powdered cumin

Garnish individual servings with cilantro leaves.

Serving idea: Serve with Dill Potato Bread.

Udon Vegetable Soup

Nice mixture of vegetables with unusual noodles.

Preparation time: 25 minutes
Cooking time: 20 – 30 minutes

Serves: 6 – 8
Autumn, Winter

Sauté in a pot until onions are golden:

¼ cup sunflower oil
1 medium onion, minced
1 clove garlic, peeled and minced

Add:

1 carrot, peeled and cut into half rounds
2 cups bok choy, sliced
1" fresh ginger, peeled and minced
1 cup green cabbage, minced
1 cup broccoli florets, cut into small pieces
1 cup mushrooms, sliced

Sauté for 5 minutes and add:

6 cups water

Cook until vegetables are soft (about 20 – 30 minutes). Add:

1 pound firm tofu, cut into ¼" cubes

While soup is cooking, break into thirds:

8 ounces Udon noodles

Cook according to the package instructions. Add cooked noodles to soup.

Blend in blender:

1½ tablespoons sesame oil
3 tablespoons raw tahini
1 tablespoon mellow miso
1 tablespoon tamari or Bragg Liquid Aminos
1 cup of broth from the soup

Add blended miso mixture to soup before serving. You can warm the soup as you add miso, but be careful not to bring it to a boil. (If miso is boiled, it will lose its beneficial digestive enzymes.)

Green Bean Soup

A light, elegant, cooling soup.

Preparation time: 30 minutes — Serves: 5–6
Cooking time: 45 minutes — Spring, Summer

Sauté for approximately 5 minutes:

3 tablespoons olive oil
1 medium onion, minced
2 cloves garlic, peeled and minced

Add:

2 cups red potatoes, cut into ½" cubes
4 cups green beans, trimmed and cut into 1" pieces
2 cups fresh tomatoes, diced
4 cups water

Bring to a boil and add:

2 tablespoons vegetable broth powder

Simmer for 30–45 minutes or until vegetables are tender. Let cool for 10 minutes, then pour soup into food processor, add these ingredients and purée:

1 cup packed fresh parsley leaves
2 cloves garlic, peeled
1 teaspoon salt, or to taste
½ teaspoon black pepper, or to taste
1 tablespoons fresh lemon juice
2 teaspoons maple syrup (optional)

Serve warm or at room temperature.

Garbanzo Vegetable Soup

Golden soup with a very pleasing texture.

Preparation time: 40 minutes
Cooking time: 15 minutes
Soaking time: Overnight
Cooking beans: 45 – 60 minutes

Serves: 5 – 7
Spring, Autumn, Winter

Soak overnight in 3 cups water:
1 cup dry garbanzo beans

Drain water and add:
4 cups fresh water

Bring to a boil and simmer until soft (approximately 1 hour, or more; be sure to leave yourself time for this part).

Meanwhile, steam until soft (approximately 10 minutes):
1 fennel bulb, minced

To prepare fennel bulb, cut off fennel stalks at the point where they meet the top and sides of the bulb. Discard stalks. Also cut off the hard, circular base of the bulb. Wash and dry the bulb, then remove its dry or pulpy outer layers. Mince bulb and steam until soft.

Sauté in a separate pot for 5 minutes:
¼ cup olive oil
1 medium onion, sliced
1 yam, cut into chunks
1 carrot, peeled and cut into rounds
2 stalks celery, cut into diagonals

Stir constantly so as not to burn.

Add:
2 cups cooked garbanzo beans (or 2 cups canned garbanzo beans)
4 cups water (using leftover water from cooking the beans)

Cook for 15 minutes (or until vegetables are soft). Let cool for 10 minutes, then purée in a food processor.

Add:

remaining cooked garbanzo beans (about 1 cup)
cooked, minced, fennel bulb
½ teaspoon paprika
1 teaspoon salt or to taste

Simmer for 5 more minutes. Before serving, add:

1–2 tablespoons fresh lemon juice (optional)

Corn Bisque

Simple, soothing, and satisfying.

Preparation time: 10 minutes — Serves: 6
Cooking time: 20 minutes — Spring, Summer

Sauté in a pot until onions are soft:

4 tablespoons melted butter or sunflower oil
1 medium onion, minced
1 bay leaf

Add and cook for approximately 20 minutes until potatoes are soft:

4 cups frozen corn, thawed
1 russet potato, peeled and cubed
3 cups water

Remove bay leaf and cool for 10 minutes. Purée in a food processor or with hand blender. Place in serving container and stir in:

¼ teaspoon dried thyme
1 teaspoon salt
¼ teaspoon black pepper

Add, just before serving:

2 tablespoons fresh cilantro, whole leaves

Miso Soup

Western version of traditional Japanese miso soup.

Preparation time: 20 minutes
Cooking time: 25 minutes

Serves: 6
Spring, Summer, Autumn

Sauté in a pot, until golden:

2 tablespoons sesame oil
1 medium onion, minced
1 tablespoon garlic, peeled and minced

Add:

2 cups mushrooms, sliced
1½ tablespoons fresh ginger, peeled and minced
1 tablespoon rice vinegar
4 cups water or stock*

Bring to a boil and simmer for 10 minutes. Then add:

1 cup firm tofu, cubed
4 green onions, sliced into thin rounds
2 cups fresh spinach, cut into strips

Simmer for another 5 minutes.

Before serving, scoop into a bowl:

2 cups liquid from soup
3 tablespoons mellow miso

Dissolve miso and return to pot. Mix well. Taste and adjust seasoning, adding tamari or Bragg Liquid Aminos as needed. If reheating is necessary, be careful not to boil the soup once miso has been added as its beneficial enzymes will be lost.

* *To make the stock, bring to a boil:*

8 cups water
5 broccoli stems (save the florets for another dish)

Simmer for 10–15 minutes. Discard stems.

Red Lentil Soup

Yummy, light soup—easy to make and an easily digested source of protein.

Preparation time: 15 minutes
Cooking time: 45 minutes

Serves: 4
Spring, Autumn, Winter

In small pot, sauté until onions are golden (approximately 5 minutes):

3 tablespoons sunflower oil
¾ cup onion, minced
2 cloves garlic, peeled and minced

Add and sauté for 3 more minutes:

2 medium carrots, peeled and cut into quarter rounds
2 celery stalks, cut into diagonals

Add:

1 cup red lentils (rinsed 3 times)
½ teaspoons powdered cumin
1 teaspoon ground coriander
¼ teaspoon turmeric
4 cups water

Bring to a boil, lower heat and simmer for approximately 40 minutes. Stir frequently and use a flame diffuser to avoid burning. Cool for 10 minutes. Add:

2 tablespoons tamari or Bragg Liquid Aminos
½ teaspoon salt
¼ teaspoon black pepper
1 pinch cayenne

Purée in a food processor or with a hand blender. Serve warm.

Serving idea: Serve with Seasoned Spinach Salad and Plain Rice or Barley Bread.

Lentil Chile Dhal

A staple of Indian cuisine—low in fat, high in fiber and protein, easy to digest. Excellent as a soup or on top of Plain Rice and vegetables.

Preparation time: 15 minutes Serves: 4–6
Cooking time: 40 minutes All Year

Place in a pot:

1½ cups red lentils (rinse 3 times)
2 whole green chiles (canned), chopped
1 teaspoon turmeric
3 bay leaves
4½ cups water

Bring to a boil and simmer. Stir often to prevent lumps. Cover partially and cook for about 30 minutes. While lentils are cooking, place in a frying pan and sauté until onions are golden:

3 tablespoons ghee or sunflower oil
1 cup onion, minced

Add to onions and stir constantly to prevent sticking and burning:

1 cup tomatoes, minced
1 tablespoon fresh ginger, peeled and grated

Continue to sauté until tomatoes are soft. Then add 1½ teaspoons salt. Blend in blender until smooth. Mix with the cooked lentils.

In a small pan heat up:

2 tablespoon ghee or sunflower oil
1 teaspoon mustard seeds
1 teaspoon cumin seeds
1 teaspoon fennel seeds

When mustard seeds start to pop, add:

¼ teaspoon dried crushed red chile pepper

When chiles turn dark (20 seconds) add:

2 teaspoons fresh garlic, minced

Turn heat off and let garlic sizzle until golden (about 25 seconds). Add the mixture of spices into dhal and mix well. Add salt to taste. Garnish with cilantro leaves and serve warm.

Variation:

Instead of red lentils you can use yellow split mung, which needs to be soaked over night. (Yellow split mung can be found in health food stores.)

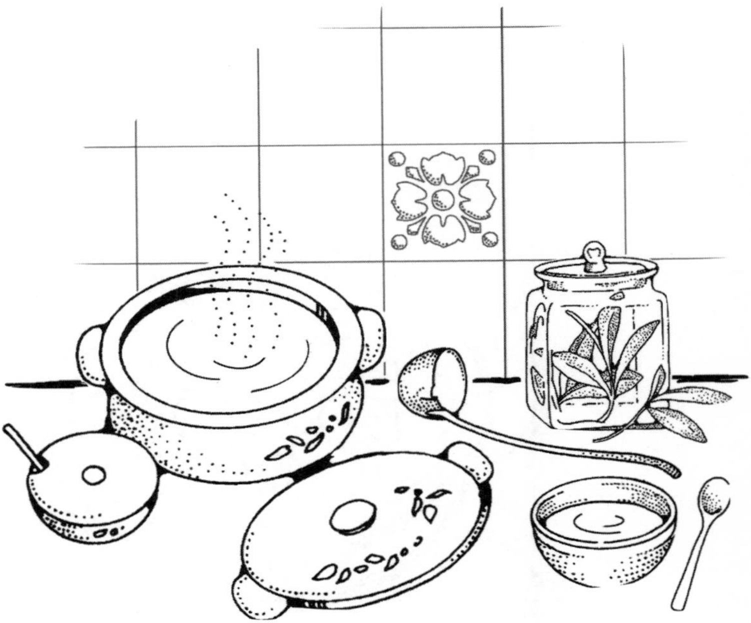

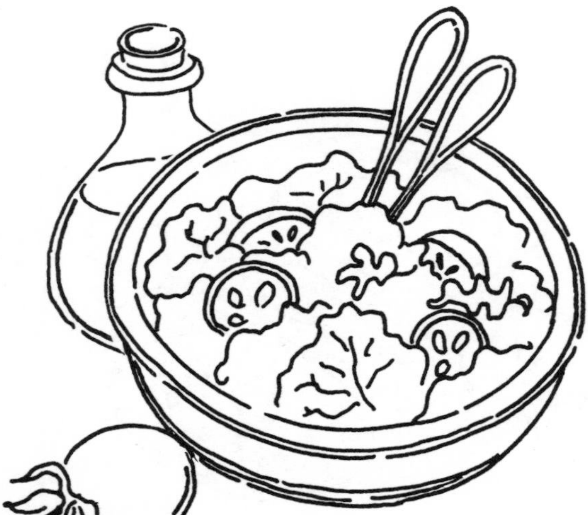

Salads and Salad Dressings

The Secret of Radiant Health and Well-Being is ...

Eating more fresh, raw food. Remember, your food consists of more than chemicals. Choose foods that are rich in life-force.

Raw Kale Salad
Sunflower Kale Salad
Radish Romaine Salad
Tomato Basil Salad
Seasoned Spinach Salad
Sweet Zucchini Salad
Potato Leek Salad
Red Pesto Pasta Salad
Lemon Ginger Dressing
Poppy Seed Dressing
Vitality Dressing
Honey Mustard Vinaigrette
Ranch Dressing
Dill Yogurt Dressing
Summer Dressing
Orange Shallot Dressing
Sesame Dressing

Raw Kale Salad

Excellent refreshment on a warm spring day.

Preparation time: 10–15 minutes
Marinating time: 1 hour
Serves: 6
Spring

Prepare the marinade by mixing in a bowl:

¼ cup olive oil
2 tablespoons fresh lemon juice
2 tablespoons tamari or Bragg Liquid Aminos
1 tablespoon sesame seeds

Wash:

1 large bunch fresh green kale

Separate the kale leaves from their stems and wash the leaves. Dry leaves thoroughly, preferably in a salad spinner. Cut the leaves into strips (see Appendix A).

Mix kale with the marinade. Cover and refrigerate for at least 1 hour before serving. (This allows kale to soften and absorb flavors.)

Sunflower Kale Salad

A creative way to enjoy leafy greens.

Preparation time: 15 minutes
Steaming time: 10 minutes
Serves: 4–5
Spring, Autumn, Winter

Wash in cold water:

1 large bunch fresh green kale

Separate the kale leaves from their stems and wash the leaves. Discard the stems (or save for soup stock or broth). Coarsely chop leaves. Steam for 10 minutes or until leaves are soft. Put kale in a salad bowl.

Sauté for 3 minutes:

¼ cup olive oil
4 green onions, minced

Add olive oil and green onions to the kale and toss together.

Mix in:

⅓ cup sunflower seeds, roasted
2 tablespoons tamari or Bragg Liquid Aminos

Radish Romaine Salad

Variation on raw green salad.

Preparation time: 15 minutes | Serves: 6 – 8 | Spring, Summer

Mix:

1 head romaine lettuce, washed, drained and cut into strips
1 cucumber, peeled, seeded, and cut into long strips*
6 radishes, cut into thin half rounds

Season with:

4 tablespoons olive oil
4 tablespoons fresh lemon juice
salt and pepper to taste

Variations:

Add 1 cup crumbled feta cheese. You can also substitute Lemon Ginger Dressing for the above seasonings.

** Cucumber preparation: Peel and cut lengthwise in half. Remove seeds and cut each half into 4 strips. Cut each strip crosswise into 3 pieces.*

Tomato Basil Salad

A cooling salad for a festive or everyday meal.

Preparation time: 25 minutes

Serves: 6
Spring, Summer

Place in a bowl:

3 large tomatoes, cut into crescents
6 mushrooms, cut into ⅛" slices
¼ cup olives, sliced
⅓ cup artichoke hearts,* quartered
¼ cup fresh parsley, minced
2 tablespoons fresh basil, minced

In a small bowl, mix dressing:

3 tablespoons red wine vinegar
6 tablespoons olive oil
1 large clove garlic, peeled and minced
2 pinches dried mustard

Pour dressing over vegetables and toss. Add, to taste:

½ teaspoon salt
¼ teaspoon black pepper

Serving idea: Good with Bulgur Garbanzo Salad.

**Use artichoke hearts packed in water, not vinegar.*

Seasoned Spinach Salad

Simple but delicious.

Preparation time: 10–15 minutes
Cooking time: 15–20 minutes

Serves: 4
All Year

Thaw and drain water from:

1 pound frozen spinach

Sauté in a skillet for 5 minutes:

3 tablespoons olive oil
4 cloves of garlic, peeled and whole
thawed spinach

Cover and let simmer on low heat for 15–20 minutes. Stir occasionally. Discard garlic cloves. Place spinach in a serving dish and add:

½ cup black olives, sliced

Serve warm.

Variations:

Add ½ cup pine nuts to sautéed spinach. You can also mix this salad with cooked basmati rice.

Sweet Zucchini Salad

Colorful accent to main course.

Preparation time: 10 minutes
Cooking time: 10 minutes

Serves: 6
All Year

Sauté for 5 minutes:

¼ cup olive oil
2 cloves garlic, peeled and minced
1 red bell pepper, cut into thin strips

Add and sauté until slightly soft:

6 zucchini, cut into rounds

Add:

2 tablespoons tamari or Bragg Liquid Aminos
2 teaspoons maple syrup
1 pinch black pepper

Serve warm or cold.

Potato Leek Salad

Hearty and filling. Nice blend of herbs.

Preparation time: 35 – 40 minutes
Cooking time: 20 – 25 minutes

Serves: 5 – 6
Spring, Autumn, Winter

Place in a pot:

5 russet potatoes, peeled and cut into chunks

Bring to a boil, then reduce heat and simmer until soft but firm. Strain and set aside.

Meanwhile, sauté until leeks are tender (approximately 10 minutes):

¼ cup sunflower oil
3 cups leeks, cut into ½" rounds
3 cloves garlic, peeled and minced

Add:

1½ teaspoons oregano
1½ teaspoons dried basil
2 teaspoons salt
¼ teaspoon black pepper

Mix the cooked potato chunks with the leeks and herbs. Serve warm.

Red Pesto Pasta Salad

A festive, colorful, new creation that everyone likes.

Preparation time: 40 minutes
Cooking time: 15 minutes

Serves: 10–12
Summer, Spring

Pour 2 cups boiling water over:

½ cup sundried tomatoes

Let soak for 15 minutes, and set aside.

Cook 1 package of Penne Pasta (16 ounces) according to package instructions. While cooking pasta, place in food processor, chop and blend lightly:

3 cloves garlic, peeled
soaked and drained sundried tomatoes (save liquid)
¼ cup liquid from tomatoes
½ teaspoon balsamic vinegar
½ teaspoon red wine vinegar
¼ teaspoon crushed dried red chile pepper
½ cup sliced olives
1 tablespoon dried thyme
1 tablespoon dried rosemary
½ cup olive oil

Place in a bowl and mix :

1 cup Parmesan, finely grated
1 cup fresh Italian parsley, chopped
3 tablespoons fresh lemon juice
1 cup sliced olives
1 teaspoon salt
cooked pasta
blended ingredients from food processor

Serve at room temperature.

Lemon Ginger Dressing

A robust, crowd-pleasing dressing that can accent any dish.

Preparation time: 40 minutes

Makes: 2½ cups
All Year

Blend in a blender until smooth:

1 cup sunflower oil
⅔ cup fresh lemon juice
6 tablespoons tamari or Bragg Liquid Aminos
⅓ cup water
2 tablespoons fresh ginger, peeled and sliced
3 tablespoons sunflower seeds
2 teaspoons dry mustard
2 cloves garlic, peeled (optional)

Keep refrigerated.

Poppy Seed Dressing

Sweet and tangy.

Preparation time: 10 minutes

Makes: 3 cups
All Year

Blend in a blender until smooth:

½ cup water
1 cup apple cider vinegar
3 tablespoons prepared Dijon mustard
⅓ medium onion, minced
1½ tablespoons poppy seeds
1½ teaspoons salt
2½ tablespoons honey
1⅓ cups oil

Keep refrigerated.

Vitality Dressing

A wonderful salad dressing, and it's also great on steamed vegetables, cooked grains, and beans. Based on a recipe contributed by Carlton Schreiner.

Preparation time: 10 minutes

Makes: 2 cups
All Year

Combine in a bowl:

2 cups sunflower or olive oil*
½ cup tamari or Bragg Liquid Aminos
2 teaspoons ground coriander
2 teaspoons powdered ginger
2 teaspoons powdered cumin
2 teaspoons dried basil
2 teaspoons dried dill weed
3 teaspoons granulated onion
4 teaspoons prepared Dijon mustard

Stir well, or pour into blender and mix on low speed for one minute.

** If using olive oil, this dressing may harden when refrigerated. Should this occur, place the container in hot water for a few minutes before serving.*

Honey Mustard Vinaigrette

A non-fat, sweet, tangy dressing.

Preparation time: 15 minutes

Makes: 2½ cups
All Year

Blend in a blender until smooth:

¼ cup natural rice vinegar
¼ cup red wine vinegar (or white wine vinegar)
½ cup fresh lemon juice
¾ cup honey
⅔ cup prepared Dijon mustard
½ teaspoon black pepper
3 tablespoons tamari or Bragg Liquid Aminos
¼ teaspoon salt
1½ teaspoons dried dill weed
1½ teaspoons Spike® seasoning

Keep refrigerated.

Ranch Dressing

A light and flavorful herbal dairy dressing.

Preparation time: 30 minutes

Makes: 2 cups
All Year

Mix all ingredients in a bowl:

1 cup plain low fat yogurt
1 cup mayonnaise
1 teaspoon dried chives
1 teaspoon dried parsley
½ teaspoon granulated garlic
½ teaspoon granulated onion
½ teaspoon powdered cumin

¼ teaspoon paprika
1 generous pinch salt
1 generous pinch black pepper

Stir well. Keep refrigerated and serve chilled.

Dill Yogurt Dressing

Good on mixed greens or Plain Rice, and as a dairy vegetable dip.

Preparation time: 10 minutes

Makes: 2½ cups
All Year

Blend in a blender until smooth:

½ cup olive oil
2 cucumbers, peeled, seeded, and sliced
½ teaspoon salt
4 tablespoons fresh dill, minced
1 dash black pepper

Fold in:

1 cup low fat yogurt, plain

Keep refrigerated and serve chilled.

Summer Dressing

A light, refreshing, green summer dressing.

Preparation time: 20 minutes

Makes: 1½ cups
Spring, Summer

Blend in a blender until smooth:

1 cup olive oil
½ cup fresh lemon juice
1 bunch fresh basil leaves
3 tablespoons prepared Dijon mustard
12 small fresh mint leaves
½ teaspoon salt
1 pinch black pepper, coarse

Tip: If refrigeration causes this dressing to harden, place the container in hot water for a few minutes before serving.

Orange Shallot Dressing

A light, slightly sweet and tangy dressing—excellent with mixed greens for a festive meal.

Preparation time: 15 minutes

Makes: 1½ cups
Spring, Summer

In blender, mix

1½ tablespoons minced shallot
½ cup fresh squeezed orange juice

While blending, slowly drizzle in:

1 cup olive oil

Blend until thickens and becomes creamy colored.

Add to blender:

½ teaspoon salt (or to taste)

¼ teaspoon black pepper
1 tablespoon fresh lemon juice
1 tablespoon honey (or less, to taste)

Serving idea: Toss with green salad and serve. Dressing is best used within 2 days.

Variation:

You can use 1 tablespoon of minced red onion instead of 1½ tablespoons minced shallot.

Sesame Dressing

A light and nutty dressing.

Preparation time: 15 minutes

Makes: ¾ cup
Spring, Summer, Autumn

Mix:

2 tablespoons balsamic vinegar
1 tablespoon orange peel, minced (optional)
1½ teaspoon Dijon mustard
½ cup vegetable broth*
2 tablespoons sesame oil
2 teaspoons roasted sesame seeds (see "Roasting Grains, Nuts & Seeds" page 106)
¼ teaspoon black pepper (or to taste)
½ teaspoon salt (or to taste)

Serving idea: Toss with green salad and serve. Best served fresh as it does not store well.

* *½ cup boiling water + 1 teaspoon vegetable broth powder*

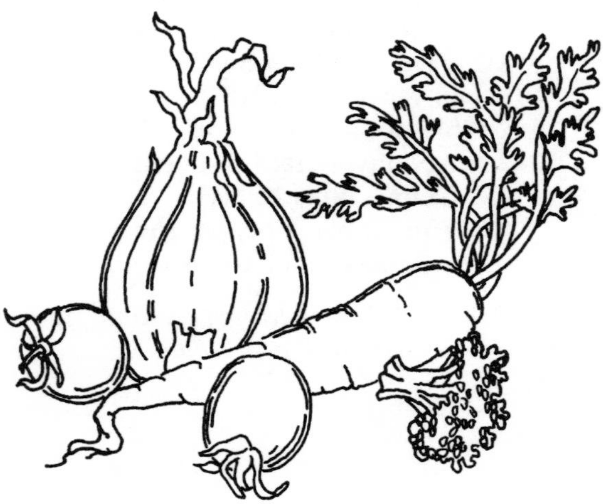

Vegetables

The Secret of Radiant Health and Well-Being is . . .

Gratitude, which opens windows to the sunlight of infinite abundance.

Yam Delight

A delightful variation on baked yams.

Preparation time: 15 minutes
Baking time: 20 – 30 minutes
Preheat oven to 400°

Serves: 4 – 6
Autumn, Winter

Simmer in a sauce pan for 5 minutes:

¼ cup sunflower oil
1 tablespoon powdered cloves
1 lemon rind, peeled and finely minced

Set aside.

Scrub well with water:

3 medium yams

Pat dry the yams and cut lengthwise into halves, then cut across each half (so you will have 4 pieces from each yam).

Strain the oil mixture and brush on yam halves on all surfaces. Place on a baking tray with the open "face" of each yam piece turned down. Bake at 400° for 20 – 30 minutes until yams are soft. Cut slits into baked yams, and drizzle some of the leftover marinade on top of the yams.

Serve warm.

Sesame Yams

Extremely easy way to create a winning side dish.

Preparation time: 10 minutes
Baking time: 30 – 40 minutes
Preheat oven to 375°

Serves: 4
Autumn, Winter

Peel and cut into 1" rounds:

3 medium yams

Mix in a bowl:

¼ cup olive oil
2 tablespoons sesame seeds

Coat yams with sesame seed mixture. Place yams on baking tray and bake at 375° for approximately 30–40 minutes or until yams are soft.

Gingered Yams

Can be served as a side dish or as a dessert.

Preparation time: 10 minutes
Baking time: 30 minutes
Preheat oven to 375°

Serves: 4
Autumn, Winter

Peel and cut into 1" rounds:

2 medium yams

Mix in a bowl:

2 tablespoons olive oil
1 tablespoon maple syrup
2 tablespoons fresh ginger juice*
½ teaspoon powdered ginger

Coat the yams with the ginger mixture. Place on a baking tray and bake approximately 30 minutes at 375°, or until yams are soft.

**To make ginger juice: Grate whole, fresh ginger root. Place a small amount at a time into your palm, and squeeze its juice into a bowl. Discard ginger pulp. Or use a garlic press to squeeze fresh ginger: Place grated, unpeeled ginger into garlic press, and squeeze juice into a bowl.*

Baked Fennel Bulbs

Delicious and filling, yet low in calories—great for weight watchers. It's a wonderful way to enjoy an unusual vegetable.

Preparation time: 20 minutes
Steaming time: 20 minutes
Baking time: 15 – 20 minutes
Preheat oven to 350°

Serves: 2 – 4
Autumn, Winter

Steam until tender, for approximately 20 minutes:

2 fennel bulbs, cut into quarters*

Place steamed fennel into a 9" glass pie dish. Mix in a separate bowl:

2 tablespoons tamari or Bragg Liquid Aminos
2 tablespoons olive oil

Pour over fennel. In a separate bowl, combine:

1 cup boiling water
1½ teaspoons powdered vegetable broth
2 tablespoons ghee or butter
5 tablespoons whole wheat pastry flour

Mix well and add:

tender feathery leaves from center of fennel stem

Pour broth mixture on fennel and bake at 350° for 15 – 20 minutes until bulbs are golden brown.

**How to cut fennel: Wash entire vegetable. Remove tender feathery leaves from the middle portion of the stalks and set leaves aside. Cut off fennel stalks at the point where they meet the top and sides of the bulb. Discard stalks. Also trim the hard circular base of bulb, leaving ⅛" of the base to keep bulb intact during cooking. Remove dry or pulpy outer layers, and cut bulb lengthwise into quarters.*

Colorful Baked Vegetables

Original and simple way to enjoy vegetables. Good with Hummus and Plain Rice.

Preparation time: 15 – 20 minutes
Baking time: 30 – 45 minutes
Preheat oven to 375°

Serves: 4
Autumn, Winter

Mix in a bowl:

¼ cup olive oil
1 teaspoon salt
¼ cup fresh lemon juice
¼ teaspoon black pepper

Add to marinade:

3 celery stalks, cut into ½" diagonals
2 carrots, peeled and cut in chunks
3 green onions, chopped (optional)
4 whole cloves garlic, peeled (optional)
1 yam, peeled and cut into ½" cubes

Coat vegetables thoroughly. Spread vegetables on baking tray and bake at 375° for 30–45 minutes, making sure vegetables are soft inside and crispy outside.

Note: When multiplying the recipe for larger quantities, the oil does not need to be increased proportionally. For example, if tripling the recipe, double the oil.

Tahini Eggplant

Tastes like Stroganoff—and it's non-dairy. Very popular.

Preparation time: 40 minutes
Cooking time: 10–15 minutes
Serves: 6
Autumn, Winter

Steam (or bake at 350°) until soft:

1 eggplant, cubed

Sauté in a pot or large skillet until onions are golden:

2 tablespoons sunflower oil
2 tablespoons olive oil
2 cups onions, minced
3 cloves garlic, peeled and minced

Add and sauté for 5 minutes:

2 cups mushrooms, sliced
cooked eggplant

Mix in:

1 teaspoon dried dill weed
1 teaspoon powdered cumin
1½ teaspoons salt
¼ teaspoon black pepper
1 pinch cayenne

Set aside. Blend in blender:

3 tablespoons raw tahini
3 tablespoons water
juice of one lemon

Add blended ingredients to sautéed vegetables and mix well. Add salt and pepper to taste.

Garnish with:

¼ cup fresh parsley, minced

Optional: Add ¼ cup red bell pepper, cubed (more flavorful if sautéed in olive oil first).

Serving idea: Great when accompanied by Rosemary Olive Bread.

Roasted Eggplant with Balsamic Dressing

A great, easy-to-make side dish.

Preparation time: 20 minutes
Baking time: 45 minutes
Preheat oven to 350°

Serves: 6
Spring, Summer

Wash and slice into ⅜" rounds:

1 large eggplant

Brush both sides of eggplant with olive oil. Place eggplant slices on baking tray in a single layer. Bake for 45 minutes at 350° until slightly browned. While eggplant is baking, mix:

2 tablespoons balsamic vinegar
¼ cup olive oil
1 teaspoon salt
1 teaspoon black pepper

Place baked eggplant on serving tray. Drizzle dressing over eggplant slices. Garnish with:

¼ cup fresh basil, thinly sliced
fresh tomatoes, sliced or quartered

Serve warm or at room temperature.

Serving idea: Serve with Focaccia and Radish Romaine Salad.

Mexican Vegetables

Colorful, hearty and spicy.

Preparation time: 35 minutes
Cooking time: 15 – 20 minutes

Serves: 6
All Year

Sauté in a pot for 5 minutes:

- **2 tablespoons sunflower oil**
- **2 cups onions, cut into crescents**
- **2 cloves garlic, peeled and minced**
- **1½ cups zucchini, cut into rounds**

Add:

- **1½ cups red or green bell peppers, cubed**
- **2 cups canned diced tomatoes (be sure to save the juice)**
- **2 cups frozen corn, thawed**
- **2 cups cooked kidney beans (canned or fresh)**
- **1 tablespoon powdered cumin**
- **1 tablespoon ground coriander**
- **1½ tablespoons chile powder**
- **1 large pinch cayenne**
- **2 teaspoons salt (or to taste)**

Mix all ingredients. Simmer until vegetables are soft. Thin with juice from the tomatoes, until it is the consistency of stew.

Serving ideas: Serve with Poppy Seed Cornbread and Mexican Rice. For a dairy option, you can serve with grated cheese and sour cream.

Variation:

For a spicier dish, add your favorite salsa to the stew.

Pad Thai

Variation on a favorite dish from Thailand.

Preparation time: 40 minutes
Cooking time: 20 minutes
Serves: 5
All Year

Mix:

5 tablespoons tamari or Bragg Liquid Aminos
2 tablespoons peanut butter
2 garlic cloves, peeled, and minced (or 2 teaspoons garlic powder)
1 tablespoon fresh ginger, peeled and grated (or 2 teaspoons ginger powder)
1 tablespoon brown sugar or honey

Blend in a blender or food processor. Put in a bowl and add:

1 pound firm tofu (not silken), cubed

Set aside, stirring occasionally.

Mix together:

8 green onions, cut into rounds (green and white parts)
14 mushrooms, sliced or quartered
½ serrano chile, seeded and minced (add more to taste, or use 1–2 teaspoons dried red chile pepper)
4 cups fresh vegetables cut into bite size pieces (e.g., snow peas, red bell peppers, broccoli, cauliflower, carrots or any combination)

Stir-fry small amounts of vegetables at a time in a small amount of sunflower or peanut oil.

Cook according to package directions:

8 ounces pasta (e.g., fettuccine or linguine) or bean thread noodles (available at Asian markets)

In a large bowl, combine tofu mixture, stir-fried vegetables, cooked pasta or noodles and:

2½ tablespoons peanuts, roasted

Serve hot or cold. If serving hot, heat the entire mixture thoroughly.

Thai Stir Fry

Excellent main dish from Ananda's EarthSong Café. *A real crowd pleaser.*

Preparation time: 30 minutes
Cooking time: 15 minutes

Serves 4
Spring, Summer, Autumn

Place in blender and blend until creamy:

1 tablespoon fresh ginger, peeled and diced
3 cloves garlic, peeled
1 tablespoon sunflower oil
1 tablespoon sesame oil
¼ cup honey
¼ cup rice vinegar
⅓ cup peanut butter
⅓ cup tamari
pinch cayenne (increase to make hot and spicy)

Lightly steam:

1 head broccoli florets, cut into bite size pieces

Cook 1 package (8.8 ounces) udon noodles according to directions on package.

While noodles are cooking, stir fry or sauté for 3–5 minutes:

2 tablespoons sunflower oil
1 red bell pepper, cut in strips then halved

Add small amount of sauce and then add:

2 cups sliced mushrooms
1½ cup shredded red cabbage
steamed broccoli florets

Cook for about 10 minutes until vegetables are slightly soft yet crisp.

Add remainder of sauce.

Drain noodles. Add cooked noodles to vegetables and stir fry until hot.

Serving idea: Excellent with mixed green salad tossed with Sesame Dressing.

Variation:

Substitute 4 raw zucchini (cut into half rounds) for 1 head steamed broccoli florets.

Sautéed Turnips

This sweet and salty side dish will keep you returning for seconds.

Preparation time: 5 minutes
Cooking time: 15 – 20 minutes

Serves: 5 – 6
Autumn, Winter

Peel and cut into thin half moons:

3 medium turnips (peeling is not necessary if turnips are fresh)

Sauté turnips for 3 minutes in:

2 – 3 tablespoons sesame oil

Sprinkle with salt and cover. Simmer for an additional 10–15 minutes. The turnips will "sweat" and cook in their own juices (the salt draws the juice out) bringing out their sweetness. If needed, add a little water, cover and simmer until turnips are soft. Turn heat off and drizzle tamari or Bragg Liquid Aminos over turnips. Place in a bowl and sprinkle with fresh parsley before serving.

Vegetable Empanada

A vegetarian version of a typical meat and vegetable pie from Spain.

Preparation time: 40 minutes
Baking time: 40 minutes
Preheat oven to 375°

Serves: 4 – 6 (makes one 9" pie)
Spring, Autumn, Winter

Mix and sauté in a small pot for 5 minutes:

4 – 6 tablespoons olive oil
1 cup onions, cut into crescents
1 cup carrots, peeled and cut into half rounds
1 cup turnips, cut into thin quarters, or 1 cup peas

Then add:

1 cup frozen chopped spinach (thawed and drained)
1 tablespoon paprika
1 teaspoon salt

Cover pot and simmer for 10 minutes. Turn heat off and set aside.

For the bottom and top crusts, combine:

2¼ cups whole wheat pastry flour
1 egg
¼ cup olive oil
½ teaspoon salt
½ cup cold water

Mix together with a wooden spoon until dough forms. Divide the dough: ⅔ for the bottom and ⅓ for the top. Roll dough thin and place in oiled 9" pie dish. Pat dough down lightly on the bottom and sides. Prick dough with a fork. Spoon in the vegetable filling. Cover with top crust (rolled out to thin round size that would cover top), and make small slits in top crust to let steam out. Brush top crust with egg-wash (see page 159). Cover with foil and bake for 30 minutes at 375°. Remove foil and bake for another 10 minutes.

Serving idea: Serve with Plain Quinoa and Tahini Sauce.

Burdock Root and Carrots

A little known root vegetable in a new variation as a nutritious and colorful side dish.

Preparation time: 5 minutes
Cooking time: 20 minutes
Serves: 2
Autumn, Winter

Scrub thoroughly in water or peel, then cut into half rounds:

1 burdock root*, 15" long (approximately ½ cup)

Place in a skillet and sauté for 2 minutes:

1–2 tablespoons sesame oil
2 tablespoons white sesame seeds

Add and sauté burdock for 3 minutes. Then add and sauté for an additional 3 minutes:

1 medium carrot, peeled and cut into diagonals

Add:

½ cup water

Cover and simmer for approximately 10 minutes or until water is absorbed. Drizzle tamari or Bragg Liquid Aminos over vegetables. Cover and let sit for 5–10 minutes. Add more tamari or Bragg Liquid Aminos to taste if needed.

** Burdock root is available at Asian grocery stores and some health food stores.*

Moroccan Stew

Wonderful mixture of vegetables and spices. A delight for the taste buds, and beautiful to look at.

Preparation time: 35 minutes
Soaking time: Overnight
Cooking beans: 60 – 90 minutes
Cooking time: 25 minutes

Serves: 6
Autumn, Winter

Soak overnight in 1½ cups water:
½ cup dry garbanzo beans

Drain and rinse beans. Place beans in pot with fresh water 3"–4" above beans. Bring to a boil and simmer until soft (approximately 60–90 minutes). Add water if needed.

Meanwhile, steam together until soft, yet crisp (approximately 10 minutes):
1 cup carrots, peeled and cut into half rounds
2 cups yams, peeled and cubed

Steam separately, until soft:
1½ cups eggplant, cubed (peeled or unpeeled)

Set aside both batches of steamed vegetables, keeping them separate.

Sauté in a large pot until onions are translucent:
1½ tablespoons olive oil
1½ cups onions, cut into crescents
1 clove garlic, peeled and minced

Mix and add to onions and garlic:
1 teaspoon powdered cumin
1 teaspoon turmeric
1 teaspoon paprika
1 teaspoon salt
¼ teaspoon ground cinnamon
1 pinch cayenne

Add:
1 cup green bell pepper, cut into strips

Cook for 5 minutes, then add:

2 cups zucchini, cut into rounds

Cook for 5 minutes, then add steamed carrots, yams, and eggplant. Then add cooked garbanzo beans and:

1 cup tomato, cubed
⅓ cup raisins

Simmer and stir often until all vegetables are soft. (If possible, use a flame diffuser to avoid burning.) Before serving stir in:

1–2 tablespoons honey

Garnish with roasted sliced almonds and fresh cilantro.

Note: Add tomato juice or water if more liquid is needed. You can also substitute canned garbanzo beans for dried, cooked ones.

Serving ideas: Serve on Plain Rice or whole wheat couscous with Raita.

Baked Parsnips

Baking brings out the sweetness in this vegetable dish. Excellent substitute for French fries.

Preparation time: 10 minutes
Baking time: 40 minutes
Preheat oven to 350°

Serves: 3
Autumn, Winter

Cut into thin diagonals:

3 parsnips (thick parts cut in half and then diagonally)

Brush with olive oil, then sprinkle with salt and bake at 350° for approximately 30 minutes or until soft.

Serving idea: After baking sprinkle on parsnips:

1½ tablespoons white or black sesame seeds, roasted

Stuffed Zucchini

Creative and tasty main dish.

Preparation time: 1 hour
Baking time: 15 – 20 minutes
Preheat oven to 350°

Serves: 4 – 5
Spring, Summer

Bring to a boil:
1½ cups water

Add:
½ cup white basmati rice

Bring to boil again, then simmer until water is absorbed and rice is cooked (about 10 minutes). Set aside.

Meanwhile, sauté until onions are golden:
1 tablespoon sunflower oil
1 tablespoon olive oil
¾ cup onions, minced
2 cloves garlic, peeled and minced

Add:
1 teaspoon dried thyme

Set aside. Bring to a boil in a pot:
8 cups water (with pinch of salt)

Add and cook for 10 minutes:
5 whole zucchini

Drain cooking water, then run cold water over zucchini to stop the cooking process. Trim ends of the zucchini, cut them lengthwise into halves, and scoop out the inside pulp. Chop and save the pulp.

Mix cooked rice, sautéed onions, and chopped zucchini pulp. Add:
¼ cup fresh parsley, minced
½ teaspoon salt (or to taste)
¼ teaspoon black pepper

Fill zucchini with stuffing and sprinkle bread crumbs on top. Place on baking tray and drizzle with olive oil to prevent drying. Bake at 350° for 15–20 minutes.

Serving idea: Good with Aduki Bean Salad and Sweet Basil Carrots.

Cilantro Beets

Really brings out the natural flavor of beets.

Preparation time: 10 minutes
Baking time: 45–60 minutes

Serves: 4–6
Spring, Autumn, Winter

Preheat oven to 350°

Place in a glass baking pan (9" x 13" works well):

4 medium beets, cut in half (lengthwise)
½ inch water

Cover with foil and bake at 350° for 45–60 minutes until soft. Let beets cool slightly, then peel them and cut into cubes or slices. (After baking, the skin becomes soft and is easy to peel off with your fingers.)

Pour on top of the beets the following mixture of:

1½ tablespoons olive oil
1½ tablespoons fresh lemon juice
1 packed tablespoon whole, fresh cilantro leaves without stems

Serve warm or cold.

Roasted Potatoes

A creative variation on French fries.

Preparation time: 15 minutes
Baking time: 30 minutes
Preheat oven to 425°

Serves: 4–6
All Year

Wash, scrub and dry:

4 medium baking potatoes

Cut each potato into 8–10 wedges.

In large bowl, toss potatoes with:

2 tablespoons olive oil

Mix:

1 teaspoon salt
½ teaspoon black pepper
½ teaspoon paprika
½ teaspoon garlic powder (optional)

Toss seasonings with potatoes. Spread potatoes on baking sheet in a single layer. Bake approximately 30 minutes until potatoes are golden brown, crisp on the outside and soft on the inside. Turn potatoes once after 15 minutes. Adjust seasonings to taste.

Variations:

1. Substitute red skinned potatoes for baking potatoes. For seasonings, instead of paprika and garlic powder, use:

1 tablespoon dried rosemary
1½ teaspoons dried thyme
2 cloves garlic, peeled and minced (optional)

2. Use:

3 baking potatoes, cut into wedges or cut into 1" cubes
3 carrots, peeled and cut into half lengthwise and crosswise

Variations (cont.):

Mix with:

3 tablespoons olive oil
¾ cup fresh parsley, minced
salt and black pepper to taste

Bake as above. After baking sprinkle with:

¼ cup fresh parsley, minced

Herbed Vegetables

Excellent with Hummus and Plain Rice.

Preparation time: 25 minutes
Marinating time: 20 minutes
Baking time: 10 minutes

Serves: 6–8
All Year

Steam until crisp and tender (approximately 8–10 minutes):

1 head cauliflower florets, cut into small pieces
2 medium carrots, peeled and cut into half rounds
2 cups green beans, cut in halves

While vegetables are steaming, mix in a bowl for marinade:

⅓ cup olive oil
½ teaspoon dried basil
½ teaspoon dried oregano
4 tablespoons fresh lemon juice
1 teaspoon salt
1 pinch black pepper

Mix steamed vegetables with marinade in a baking pan. Let sit for 20 minutes to absorb flavors. Bake for 10 minutes at 350°. Serve warm.

Stuffed Cabbage

Vegetarian version of a traditional favorite. Top with Tahini Sauce, Sweet Tomato Sauce, or Lemon Tomato Sauce.

Preparation time: 45 minutes
Baking time: 15 – 20 minutes
Preheat oven to 350°

Serves: 6 – 8
Autumn, Winter

Bring to a boil:
2 cups water

Add:
⅔ cup rice or millet

Bring to boil again, then simmer until water is absorbed and grain is cooked. Set aside.

Sauté until onions are golden brown:
2 tablespoons sunflower oil
1 medium onion, minced

Add and sauté for 5 minutes:
2 medium carrots, peeled and cut into quarter rounds
2 celery stalks, cut into diagonals

Stir in, cover and simmer for 5 minutes:
1½ tablespoons juice of grated ginger*
¼ cup roasted sunflower seeds or walnuts
¼ cup fresh parsley, minced
3 tablespoons tamari or Bragg Liquid Aminos

Mix in a large bowl:
sautéed vegetables and 2 cups cooked grain

Set aside. Cook in 8 cups boiling water with 1 teaspoon salt:
10 green or red cabbage leaves (use more leaves if they are small)

** Grate ginger root, place small amount at a time into your palm, and squeeze juice into a bowl. Discard ginger pulp. Or use a garlic press to squeeze fresh ginger: place grated, unpeeled ginger in garlic press and squeeze juice into a bowl.*

Cook until the leaves are slightly tender. Remove leaves from water and let them cool in a bowl. Remove the hard part at bottom of each leaf, where it was connected to the core (cut out a small triangle shape).

Divide the filling into 10 equal parts. Spoon one part into the center of each leaf. Fold in the side edges to cover the filling. Bring bottom edge to meet the top to create a "roll." You can use toothpicks to secure the edges. Place the cabbage rolls on an oiled baking tray. Bake at 350° for 15–20 minutes or until slightly browned.

Leftover cabbage can be steamed, minced, and mixed into the leftover stuffing.

Tip: Before cooking the grains, you may wish to roast them in a dry skillet, stirring gently to prevent burning. Continue roasting until there is a nutty aroma. After roasting, cook grains according to recipe.

Variations for stuffing:

Sauté:

2 tablespoons sunflower oil
1 medium onion, minced
1 medium carrot, peeled and grated
½ pound firm (not silken) tofu, cubed
2 tablespoons tamari or Bragg Liquid Aminos
2 teaspoons dried dill weed
¼ cup fresh parsley, minced
2 tablespoons sesame seeds
salt to taste

Or sauté:

2 tablespoons sunflower oil
1 medium onion, minced
2 cloves garlic, peeled and minced
½ cup mushrooms, sliced
2 cups eggplant, cubed and steamed
1 teaspoon dried dill weed
¼ cup fresh parsley, minced
1 teaspoon salt (or to taste)
1 pinch black pepper

Vegetable Pasties

Delicious and non-dairy—very light and tastes great.

Preparation time: 1 hour
Baking time: 25 – 30 minutes
Preheat oven to 350°

Serves: 7 (makes 14 small pasties)
Spring, Summer, Autumn

Mix together in a bowl:

4 cups whole wheat pastry flour
1 teaspoon salt
¼ teaspoon dried thyme (optional)
¼ teaspoon dried sage (optional)
½ cup sunflower oil, or butter (melted)

Add gradually approximately:

1 cup ice water

until the mixture forms a non-sticky, one-piece dough. Cover with plastic wrap and set aside. Then sauté for approximately 5 minutes:

4 tablespoons sunflower oil
1 small onion, minced
1 carrot, peeled and cut into quarter rounds
1 cup broccoli florets, cut into small pieces
2 small zucchini, cut into half rounds
1 potato, boiled and cubed
1 cup mushrooms, sliced

Add:

1 teaspoon dried basil
1 teaspoon dried oregano
1 teaspoon salt
¼ teaspoon black pepper

In a separate bowl, mix:

½ cup cool water
1 tablespoon arrowroot powder

Add this mixture to the sautéed vegetables and cook until vegetables are soft, stirring frequently.

Roll dough until it is thin, then cut into 14 rounds. (If you have a 32-ounce yogurt container, use it for cutting the rounds.) Place 2–4 tablespoons of sautéed vegetables on half of each round. Brush water on edges of rounds (for sticking) and fold over the empty half of the round. Seal by pinching edges together. Place pasties on a baking tray and prick top with fork to release steam. Bake at 350° for 25–30 minutes. Immediately upon removing from oven, brush with oil or butter.

Use Tahini Sauce or Mushroom Gravy as a topping.

Serving idea: Serve with green salad and Maple Sesame Tofu.

Vegetable Medley

Great alternative to mashed potatoes.

Preparation time: 15 minutes
Cooking time: 15–20 minutes

Serves: 4
Autumn, Winter

Place in a pot with 1 cup water:

2 potatoes, peeled and cut into cubes
1 carrot, peeled and cut into cubes
1 turnip, peeled and cut into cubes

Bring water to a boil, then simmer until vegetables are soft (approximately 15–20 minutes). Pour off any remaining water. Add:

2 tablespoons olive oil
1 teaspoon salt
1 pinch black pepper
¼ cup fresh parsley, minced

Mix together and serve warm.

Veggie Paté

A delicious main course for a festive meal.

Preparation time: 35 minutes
Baking time: 50 – 60 minutes
Preheat oven to 350°

Serves: 6 – 8
Makes: 1 loaf pan
All Year

Place in food processor:

1 cup sunflower seeds

Pulse until chopped coarsely. Mix in a large bowl:

¾ cup onion, minced
3 cloves garlic, peeled and minced

Add processed sunflower seeds to the onion mixture. Add:

1 large potato peeled and grated
½ cup whole wheat flour
¼ cup nutritional yeast
1½ tablespoons fresh lemon juice
¼ cup sunflower oil
¼ cup water
2 teaspoon dried thyme
2 teaspoon dried basil
2 teaspoon dried sage
½ teaspoon salt
½ teaspoon black pepper
1 tablespoon Dijon mustard

Mix until well combined. Pour into oiled 9" x 5" (or 6" x 10") loaf pan. Cover with foil and bake at 350° for 30 minutes. Uncover and continue baking 20 – 30 minutes until golden on top.

Serving ideas: Serve with Apricot Dijon Sauce or Golden Gravy. Sprinkle minced parsley on Veggie Paté slices.

Vegetable Wraps

Ready-made whole wheat tortillas filled with seasoned vegetables.

Preparation time: 20 minutes
Cooking time: 35 minutes

Serves: 6
Spring, Autumn, Winter

Preheat oven to 375°

Steam for 10 minutes:

1 head cauliflower cut into bite sized pieces (approximately 5 cups)

Add:

1½ cups frozen peas

Steam for an additional 5 minutes. Place steamed cauliflower and peas in a bowl, add and toss to mix:

1 tablespoon cumin powder
1 tablespoon fresh ginger, peeled and grated
2 teaspoons curry powder
1½ teaspoons salt
3 tablespoons fresh lemon juice
2 tablespoons fresh cilantro, minced
pinch cayenne

Divide into 6 portions. Place one tortilla on work space. Brush lightly with olive oil. Place one portion of vegetable mix in center of tortilla. Fold left side and right side of tortilla toward middle, then fold top and bottom to the center. Place on a baking sheet, seam side down. Repeat process with remaining tortillas. Brush top of wraps with olive oil. Bake at 375° for 15–20 minutes until crisp and golden.

Serving idea: Serve with Sweet Tomato Sauce, Indian Herbed Rice and Date Raisin Chutney.

Nori Rolls

A vegetarian version of sushi: rice and vegetables wrapped in seaweed sheets. A creative delight, nutritious, filling, and delicious.

Preparation time: 45 minutes
Cooking time: 30 – 35 minutes

Makes: 4 nori rolls
(20 – 24 pieces)
All Year

Bring to a boil:

4 cups water
1⅓ cups short grain brown rice

Reduce heat and cover. Simmer until all water is absorbed and rice is cooked and sticky. Let sit and cool for 10 minutes. (You will have about 4 cups of cooked rice.)

Meanwhile steam until al dente:

1 carrot, peeled and cut lengthwise, into ¼" thick strips.
1 red bell pepper cut into thin strips

Place each vegetable in a separate bowl.

Prepare and set in separate bowls:

1 cucumber peeled and cut lengthwise, into ¼" thick strips
3 tablespoons roasted sesame seeds

Unwrap:

4 sheets of toasted sushi nori*

If you have a bamboo sushi mat, lay 1 sheet of nori on it. Otherwise, you can work on a counter top or a cutting board and roll up the nori with your hands. Put out a small bowl of cold water to wet your hands and keep the rice from sticking to them as you work.

Place on the center of the nori sheet:

1 cup of cooked rice

Wet your hands and pat the rice evenly leaving 1" space at the top and bottom edges of the sheet. Sprinkle 1 tablespoon of sesame seeds on rice. Arrange cucumber, carrot and red bell pepper strips horizontally, in 2 or 3 rows lined up with bottom line (close to you) of rice. Moisten lightly top edge of nori (far from you) with water, using your fingers. Then tuck the edge close to you, and roll up the rice with the bamboo mat and press firmly to keep a uniform shape and size. When you come to the end of the rice allow the pressure of the roll to seal the edges. Repeat with other nori sheets. Slice each nori roll with a sharp knife into 5–6 round pieces. Serve with Dipping sauce, Miso Soup and pickled ginger.*

Variation:

Add blanched spinach leaves, avocado, jicama, (or any vegetables you like) to wrap in your nori.

** Toasted sushi nori and pickled ginger can be found in health food stores and Asian grocery stores.*

Sweet Basil Carrots

A simple way to add elegance to carrots.

Preparation time: 10 minutes — Serves: 6–8
Steaming time: 15 minutes — All Year

Steam until tender, yet crisp:

6 medium carrots, peeled and cut into diagonals

Mix in a bowl:

3 tablespoons olive oil
1 tablespoon maple syrup or honey
1 tablespoon fresh basil, minced, or 1 teaspoon dried basil

Pour marinade over steamed carrots, and coat carrots before serving. Serve warm.

Vegetables in Coconut Curry Sauce

Steamed vegetables folded into curried coconut sauce. Award-winning recipe from Ananda's EarthSong Café.

Preparation time: 20 minutes
Cooking time: 50 minutes
Serves: 6 – 8 people
All Year

Steam vegetables separately until al dente:

1 head of cauliflower florets (about 4 cups)
2 medium carrots, peeled and cut into half rounds
2 zucchini, cut into rounds
1 red bell pepper, cut into half strips
1 cup frozen peas

Set aside.

Meanwhile heat in a medium pot:

¼ cup sunflower oil or peanut oil
1 tablespoon mustard seeds

When seeds start to pop, add and sauté until onion is translucent:

1 medium onion, minced
2 tablespoons garlic, minced
¼ teaspoon dried crushed red chile pepper

Add spices and mix and cook for 3 minutes on low heat:

2 tablespoons ground coriander
1 teaspoon turmeric
1 teaspoon curry powder
1 teaspoon salt
½ teaspoon powdered cumin
½ teaspoon ground cardamom
¼ teaspoon cinnamon
pinch ground cloves

Add and simmer (do not boil):

2 cups of coconut milk (1-14oz. can of pure coconut milk)

Fold in:

steamed vegetables
1 tablespoon honey (optional)

Serve with Plain Rice, Cucumber Raita, and Lentil Chile Dhal.

Walnut Balls

A delicious substitute for meat balls.

Preparation time: 35 minutes
Baking time: 45 minutes
Preheat oven 350°

Makes: 20 balls
All Year

Grind in food processor in succession:

1 cup whole walnuts
¾ cup onion, minced
1 clove garlic, peeled
1 stalk celery, without leaves

Combine in a bowl:

2 eggs
3 tablespoons fresh parsley, minced
1 cup bread crumbs
1 teaspoon salt

Add ground ingredients to bowl with eggs and bread crumbs mixture. Add more bread crumbs or nuts if needed to create firm consistency. Roll into balls 1" in diameter. Put on oiled baking sheet and bake for 30–45 minutes. Turn balls every 10–15 minutes to cook evenly and avoid sticking and burning.

Serving idea: Good with pasta and Sweet Tomato Sauce, Lemon Tomato Sauce or Tomato Pizza Sauce.

Variation:

Substitute an equal amount of sunflower seeds for the walnuts.

Greek Spinach Frittata

Based on an Italian dish, essentially a baked omelet topped with cheese. Traditionally used for picnic fare. Excellent served warm or cold.

Preparation time: 25 minutes
Baking time: 40 minutes

Serves: 6
Makes: one 9" pie
Spring, Summer, Fall

Sauté in a large pan:
⅓ cup olive oil
1 medium onion, sliced into thin crescents

Add and sauté until soft:
1 large potato peeled and sliced into quarter rounds

Add and sauté until spinach is mostly dry:
1 10-ounce package frozen spinach, thawed, drained and squeezed

Add and mix:
½ tablespoon dried dill weed
1 teaspoon salt
½ teaspoon black pepper
¼ teaspoon dried crushed red chile pepper

Place in an oiled 9" glass pie pan and press firmly. Beat:
8 eggs

Pour eggs over top of vegetables. Sprinkle evenly over top:
1 cup feta cheese, crumbled (optional)

Bake at 350° for 40 minutes or until golden. Before serving, sprinkle paprika over top.

Variation:

Instead of potato, use 1 red bell pepper cut into 1" cubes.

Serving ideas: Serve with Olive Rosemary Bread and Tomato Basil Salad.

Squash-Stuffed Potatoes

A refreshing variation on stuffed potatoes.

Preparation time: 35 minutes
Baking time: 40 – 50 minutes
Preheat oven to 350°

Serves: 6 – 8
Spring, Autumn, Winter

Scrub, wash, and dry:

6 russet potatoes

Coat potatoes with olive oil. Prick with fork and place on baking tray. Bake at 350° for 30–40 minutes or until soft.

While potatoes are baking, peel, seed, and cube:

2 small (or 1 medium) butternut squash

Steam squash until soft.

When potatoes are cooked, cut in half. Use a spoon to scoop out the pulp, making sure to leave a thin layer of pulp to protect skin from tearing. Mash potato pulp and steamed squash together.

Add to the potato-squash mixture:

1 teaspoon powdered cumin
3 tablespoons olive oil
2 teaspoons salt
1 tablespoon dried chives
2 teaspoons fresh lemon juice (optional)
black pepper or cayenne to taste (optional)

Brush the inner layer of empty potato shells with olive oil (to prevent drying out when baking). Put squash mixture into empty potato shells (12 halves) and bake for 10 minutes at 350°.

After baking, sprinkle with olive oil and paprika and decorate with a sprig of parsley. Serve with butter or olive oil on the side for added moisture.

Dill Butternut Squash

Creative and refreshingly different.

Preparation time: 20 minutes
Baking time: 40 minutes
Preheat oven to 350°

Serves: 3 – 4
Autumn, Winter

Peel, seed, and cut into long strips* (3" long by ½" thick):

1 medium butternut squash

Place on baking tray and drizzle with olive oil to coat the squash strips. Bake approximately 40 minutes, making sure squash is soft.

In the meantime, sauté until onions are golden brown:

2 tablespoons sunflower oil
1 small onion, minced

Add:

½ teaspoon dried dill weed
¼ teaspoon black pepper

Mix with squash strips after they have been baked. Garnish with sprigs of fresh parsley. Serve warm.

** Butternut squash preparation: Cut in half, crosswise, and peel. Then cut each piece in half, lengthwise, and scoop out the seeds. Cut the pieces of squash into strips.*

Baked Zucchini

Light and tasty variation on a warm-weather favorite.

Preparation time: 15 – 20 minutes
Marinating time: 30 – 60 minutes
Baking time: 30 minutes
Preheat oven to 350°

Servings: 6
Spring, Summer

Mix in a bowl:

- **⅓ cup tamari**
- **⅓ cup olive oil**
- **3 cloves garlic, peeled and minced**
- **⅓ cup fresh lemon juice**

Add:

- **10 small zucchini, cut into quarter rounds**

Marinate for 30–60 minutes.

Spread on baking pan (9" x 13" works well). Bake at 350° for 30 minutes.

Remove from oven, place in a bowl, and mix in:

- **⅓ cup fresh parsley, minced**

Serving idea: This is a nice side dish with Plain Rice and Pinto Beans Italiano.

Stuffed Mushrooms

Rich and delicious appetizer.

Preparation time: 25 minutes
Baking time: 20 minutes
Preheat oven to 350°

Serves: 8
All Year

Sauté until onions are translucent:

2 tablespoons melted ghee or butter
½ cup onions, minced

Set aside. Then blend in food processor until minced:

¼ cup walnuts
20 mushroom stems (set caps aside for stuffing)

Combine in a bowl the sautéd onions, walnut mixture, and:

¼ cup bread crumbs

Add:

1½ tablespoons tamari or Bragg Liquid Aminos
1 pinch salt
1 pinch black pepper

Stuff mushroom caps with this mixture. Place caps with stuffing face up on oiled baking tray. Bake at 350° for 20 minutes or until light brown.

Serve with minced parsley as garnish

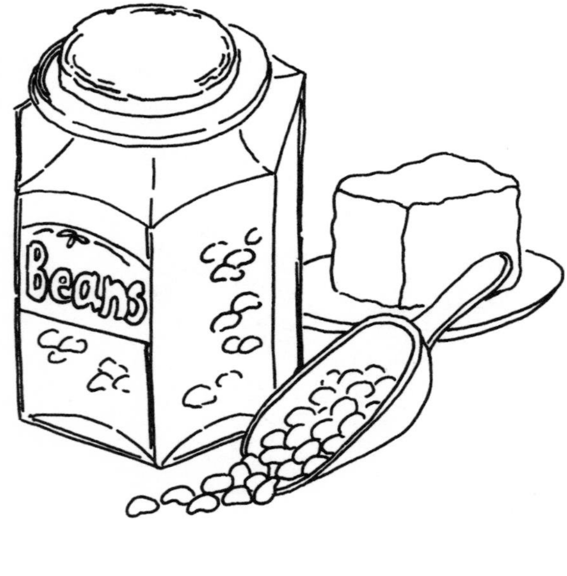

Beans

Beans and Tofu

The Secret of Radiant Health and Well-Being is . . .

Concentrating on the vital essence of what you eat. The more you make it a practice to eat consciously, the more the energy in what you eat will fill your being.

Introduction to Beans

Beans are an excellent source of protein, and an especially important protein source for vegetarians. You'll need to discover which beans are most appropriate for you, and how to prepare them so as to minimize their gas-producing qualities. When beans are well cooked and quite soft, they are easier to digest.

Sort through the dry beans carefully to remove any stones. Rinse, then soak them overnight in 3 times as much water as beans. (Note: red lentils and green split peas do not require soaking.)

Tip: If you are unable to soak the beans overnight, place the beans in a pot and cover them with water 3"–4" above beans. Bring to a boil, cover, and simmer for 5 minutes. Turn off heat and let beans soak in hot water, covered, for 2 hours.

Cooking Beans

Drain and rinse beans. Replace the soaking water with fresh water to a level of about 3"–4" above the beans. Bring to a boil and simmer for 1½–3 hours (depending on the type and age of bean) until beans are soft. Check periodically to see if more water is needed.

If you have a pressure cooker, it will save you time. Use 2–3 times as much water as beans in the pressure cooker. It can take from 20–30 minutes to cook the beans if you have soaked the beans overnight. Note: Do not pressure-cook lentils or split peas because they can clog the pressure release valve.

Beans should remain underwater during cooking. Salt toughens the skin of beans, so for quicker cooking, do not add salt to beans until they are done. When making bean salad, salt may be added during the last third of the cooking time—this helps keep the skins from slipping off the beans. Beans become tougher as they age—the older they are, the longer they need to cook.

While cooking beans, a foam might form on the surface. If foam appears, skim it off and discard. This foam is part of what contributes to gas. Continue cooking, adding water as needed.

Tofu Salad

Excellent, low-fat snack or side dish. Also nice for sandwiches. Great vegetarian alternative to tuna salad.

Preparation time: 15 minutes	Serves: 6
Chilling time: 30 minutes to 2 hours	Spring, Summer

Blend in a food processor until crumbled:

1 pound firm tofu (not silken)

Set aside in mixing bowl.

Then, finely chop in food processor:

1 medium carrot, peeled and cut into chunks

Mix with tofu.

Add to the tofu-carrot mixture:

1 celery stalk, minced fine by hand
3 tablespoons olive oil
3 tablespoons fresh lemon juice
3 tablespoons tamari or Bragg Liquid Aminos

Mix all ingredients together. Refrigerate for 30 minutes to 2 hours before serving to allow flavors to be absorbed.

Aduki Bean Salad

Nourishing and satisfying, with a pleasant combination of herbs.

Preparation time: 20 minutes
Soaking time: Overnight
Cooking beans: 60 – 90 minutes

Serves: 5
All Year

Soak overnight in 3 cups water:
1 cup dry aduki beans

Drain and rinse beans. Cover beans with:
6 cups fresh water.

Bring to a boil and simmer for 45 minutes. Add to beans:
1 teaspoon salt

Continue cooking beans until beans are very soft (about 45 minutes more). Note: Adding salt prevents the skins from slipping off the beans.

While beans are cooking, combine in a mixing bowl:
2 tablespoons fresh lemon juice
2 tablespoons olive oil
2 tablespoons tamari or Bragg Liquid Aminos
1½ teaspoons powdered cumin
1½ teaspoons ground coriander
2 tablespoons fresh parsley, minced
½ cup steamed green beans
¼ cup sunflower seeds, roasted (optional)

Drain beans and set aside the liquid. Mix the drained beans with the other ingredients. Taste and add more tamari or Bragg Liquid Aminos as needed. Add some saved liquid for a moister version.

Navy Bean Spread

Great on Basic Whole Wheat Bread, Rosemary Olive Bread, or pita bread.

Preparation time: 15 minutes
Soaking time: Overnight
Cooking beans: 60–90 minutes

Serves: 4–6
Makes: 2 cups
All Year

Rinse, then soak overnight in 3 cups water, or soak for 2 hours in 3 cups boiling water:

1 cup dry navy beans

Drain and rinse beans. Cover beans with:

3 cups fresh water

Bring to a boil and cook beans until they are very soft (approximately 60–90 minutes). Strain and save cooking water.

Place in a food processor and blend until smooth:

cooked beans
¼ cup water (use cooking water first, if any remains)
2 tablespoons olive oil
2 tablespoons fresh lemon juice
1 clove garlic, peeled (optional)
½ teaspoon powdered cumin
1 pinch cayenne
1 teaspoon salt (or to taste)
¼ teaspoon black pepper
1 pinch turmeric (optional, to create yellowish spread)

Add more cooking liquid (or water) for a creamier consistency.

Garnish with paprika, black olives, and fresh minced parsley or cilantro.

Variation:

Replace navy beans with garbanzo beans.

Pinto Beans Italiano

Delicious way to fix pinto beans.

Preparation time: 30 minutes
Soaking time: Overnight
Cooking beans: 90 minutes to 2 hours

Serves: 8
All Year

Rinse then soak overnight in 4½ cups water:

1½ cups dry pinto beans

Drain soaking water. Put beans in pot with:

6 cups fresh water
1 bay leaf
1 teaspoon ground coriander
1 teaspoon powdered cumin
½ teaspoon turmeric

Cook beans until very soft and mushy (approximately 1½–2 hours), adding water if needed. Remove bay leaf when beans are done.

While beans are cooking, sauté until onions are golden brown:

2 tablespoons sunflower oil
1 onion, minced

Add:

2 cups fresh tomatoes, cubed
1 tablespoon ground coriander
½ teaspoon black pepper

Combine sautéed vegetables with cooked beans in their pot, including any remaining liquid from cooking the beans. Add:

1 teaspoon salt (or to taste)

Just before serving, add:

½ cup fresh cilantro leaves, minced

Variation:

Omit turmeric, pepper, and salt, then add tamari or Bragg Liquid Aminos to sautéed vegetables.

Serving idea: Serve with Plain Rice and steamed broccoli.

Pinto Beans with Vegetables

Colorful and flavorful—nice with Plain Rice.

Preparation time: 35 minutes
Soaking time: Overnight
Cooking beans: 90 minutes to 2 hours

Serves: 6–8
All Year

Rinse then soak overnight in 4½ cups water:

1½ cups pinto beans

Drain, rinse then cover with fresh water 3"–4" above beans. Bring water to a boil and simmer with:

1 bay leaf
2 teaspoons ground coriander
2 teaspoons powdered cumin
1 teaspoon turmeric
1 sprig fresh rosemary, or 1 teaspoon dried rosemary

Cook until soft, then set aside.

Meanwhile, sauté until onions are golden:

3 tablespoons sunflower oil
2 medium onions, minced
3 cloves garlic, peeled and minced

Add:

2 carrots, peeled and minced
2 celery stalks, minced

Sauté and cover until vegetables are soft. Add:

½ teaspoon salt (or to taste)
black pepper to taste

Remove rosemary stem (if using fresh rosemary) and bay leaf from beans. Mix vegetables with the beans. Serve warm.

Garbanzo Stew

Sweet and sour flavor. Easy to make and substantial.

Preparation time: 25 minutes
Soaking time: Overnight
Cooking beans: 60–90 minutes
Cooking time: 20 minutes

Serves: 4
Spring, Autumn, Winter

Soak overnight in 1½ cups water:
½ cup garbanzo beans

Rinse beans 3–4 times. Add fresh water (3"–4" above beans) and bring to a boil. Simmer until soft (not mushy). Add 1 teaspoon salt after 1 hour of cooking. Strain and save water from cooking.

Meanwhile, sauté in a large pot until onions are golden:
1–2 tablespoons olive oil
2 cups onions, cut into crescents

Add to onions and sauté for 5 minutes:
2 cups mushrooms, sliced
3 cups broccoli florets, cut into small pieces

Add cooked garbanzos and 1 cup cooking water to onion mixture and combine thoroughly. Stir in and simmer on low heat for 5–10 minutes.
3 tablespoons fresh lemon juice
½ cup raisins
1 teaspoon paprika
1 teaspoon salt
1 pinch cayenne
¼ teaspoon black pepper

Serve with Plain Bulgur or Plain Millet.

Garbanzo Vegetable Curry

A hearty and satisfying curry.

Preparation time: 20 minutes
Soaking time: Overnight
Cooking beans: 60 – 90 minutes
Cooking time: 20 minutes

Serves: 10 – 12
Spring, Fall, Winter

Soak overnight in 5 cups water:
1½ cups garbanzo beans

Rinse beans 3 to 4 times. Add fresh water (3" – 4" above beans) and bring to a boil. Simmer until soft but not mushy.

Heat until the cumin seeds brown:
½ cup olive oil
½ cup sunflower oil
3 cloves garlic, peeled and minced
1½ tablespoons cumin seeds
¼ cup fresh ginger, finely grated

Add and sauté until the eggplant begins to soften:
2 medium eggplants, peeled and cut into bite-sized pieces

Add, cover and simmer for 10 – 15 minutes:
4 cups canned, whole tomatoes, cubed (save juice)
1 – 1½ cups juice from tomatoes
cooked chickpeas
2 10-ounce packages frozen spinach (approximately 4 cups), **thawed and pressed dry**
4 teaspoons salt
1 tablespoon garam masala
1 tablespoon curry powder
¼ teaspoon cayenne

Serve warm.

Serving idea: Serve with basmati rice and Cucumber Raita. Excellent served the next day as seasonings have a chance to blend.

Garbanzo "Croutons"

Delicious on salads or as a side dish.

Preparation time: 15 minutes
Soaking time: Overnight
Cooking beans: 60 – 90 minutes
Marinating time: 20 minutes
Baking time: 30 minutes

Serves: 6
Makes: 2½ cups
All Year

Rinse then soak overnight in 3 cups water:

1 cup garbanzo beans

Drain, rinse then add:

6 cups fresh water
1 teaspoon ground coriander
1 teaspoon powdered cumin
1 bay leaf
1 teaspoon powdered fennel
1 sprig fresh rosemary, or 1 teaspoon dried rosemary
1 stalk celery, cut into diagonals
1 carrot, peeled and cut into quarter rounds
1 small onion, minced

Bring to a boil and simmer for approximately 1½ hours or until garbanzo beans are soft.

While beans are cooking, combine in a bowl for marinade:

2 tablespoons tamari or Bragg Liquid Aminos
2 tablespoons olive oil
2 tablespoons fresh lime or lemon juice

Drain water. Discard vegetables (optional) and bay leaf. Place beans in a glass baking pan and pour tamari or Bragg Liquid Aminos marinade over beans.

Preheat oven to 350°. Let beans sit for 20 minutes to marinate. Bake for 30 minutes at 350° until beans are crisp on the outside and slightly tender on the inside. Be careful not to overbake as the beans will harden and be difficult to chew. Serve warm or at room temperature.

Variation: Substitute soybeans for garbanzo beans.

Hummus

This delicious Middle Eastern garbanzo spread is often used as a dip with vegetables or on pita bread. Excellent source of protein.

Preparation time: 20 minutes
Soaking time: Overnight
Cooking beans: 60 – 90 minutes

Serves: 5
All Year

Rinse then soak overnight in 3 cups water:

¾ cups garbanzo beans

Drain, rinse then cover with fresh water 3" – 4" above beans. Bring to boil, then reduce heat and simmer until beans are very soft (approximately 60 – 90 minutes).

Blend in food processor until smooth:

2 cups garbanzo beans—cooked or canned
⅔ cup water from cooking garbanzo beans
3 tablespoons raw tahini
2 cloves garlic, peeled (optional)
1 teaspoon salt
2 tablespoons olive oil
2 tablespoons fresh lemon juice

Add and blend for an additional minute:

2 tablespoons fresh parsley leaves
1 pinch cayenne
2 pinches paprika

Place hummus in a bowl and sprinkle olive oil on top of dish to prevent drying. You can decorate with paprika, sprigs of parsley or mint, and sliced or whole olives.

Tofu Puff Pasties

Excellent main dish when served with Mushroom Gravy. Especially nice touch for a holiday meal.

Preparation time: 45 minutes
Baking time: 15 – 20 minutes
Preheat oven to 350°

Makes: 12 small pasties (serves: 5 – 6)
All Year

Thaw:

2 sheets frozen puff pastry (one 17¼-ounce package, available in most markets)

Leave at room temperature, covered with a damp towel.

Mix together in a bowl:

1 pound firm tofu (not silken), crumbled
2 green onions, minced
2 tablespoons fresh basil, minced, or 1½ teaspoons dried basil

Add to tofu mixture:

2 tablespoons olive oil
4 tablespoons fresh lemon juice

Place in a glass pan. Sprinkle on top:

1 zucchini, cut into quarter rounds
1 ripe tomato, cubed

Bake at 350° until tomato and zucchini are soft.

Meanwhile, sauté for 3 minutes:

2 tablespoons olive oil
1 cup fresh spinach, cut into strips

Mix spinach with the baked tofu mixture and add:

1 teaspoon salt
¼ teaspoon black pepper (or to taste)

Roll out each puff pastry sheet thin enough to make 6 rounds. (If you have a 32 ounce yogurt container, it works well for creating the rounds.) Strain stuffing to remove excess liquid. (If stuffing is too moist, it will be difficult to seal pasties.) Divide the stuffing into 12 portions. Place the filling on one half of each dough round, leaving ¼" space around the edge.

Brush a small amount of water on the edge (just enough to make it sticky; too much makes it slippery), and close the pastry, pressing it together with your fingers to seal.

Pierce a hole at the top for release of steam. Brush with egg-wash or milk (see "Brushing the Surface of Yeasted Breads and Rolls," page 159) and bake on ungreased baking tray at 350° for 15–20 minutes or until golden brown.

Serving idea: For decoration, use a leaf-shaped cookie cutter to cut pieces of any leftover dough. (A maple leaf shape looks very nice.) Brush the back of each leaf with water and "stick" a leaf on the top of each pastry.

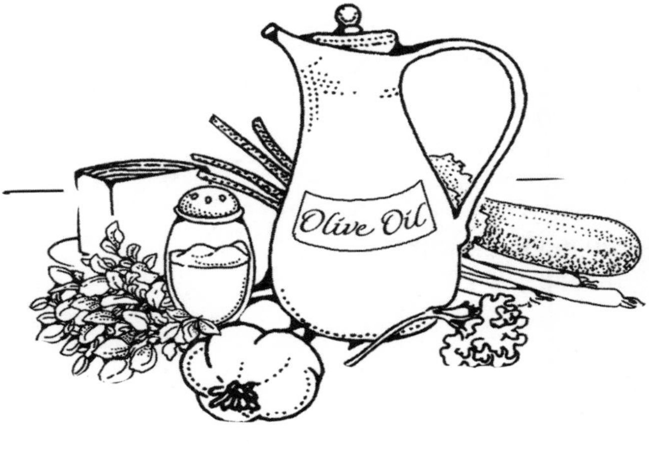

Tofu Spinach Pie

This is a non-dairy, healthy version of Greek spinach pie (spanakopitta).

Preparation time: 40 minutes
Baking time: 30 minutes
Preheat oven to 350°
Serves: 6
All Year

Mix in a bowl:

1¾ cup whole wheat pastry flour
½ teaspoon salt

Combine thoroughly with:

¼ cup sunflower oil

Add:

½ cup cold water

Mix until it forms a ball of dough. Roll and flatten dough. Place in bottom of well oiled glass 9" pie dish. Press dough with your fingers, starting from the center until it fully covers the sides of the dish. Make sure the dough is evenly distributed. Prick bottom of dough with fork. Bake for 10 minutes at 350°.

Mix together in a bowl:

1 pound firm tofu (not silken), **crumbled by hand or food processor**
4 tablespoons olive oil
2 tablespoons fresh lemon juice
2 teaspoons salt
½ teaspoon black pepper
1 teaspoon garlic powder

Set aside.

Sauté until onions are golden:

2 tablespoons sunflower oil
1 cup onions, minced

Add and sauté for 3 minutes or until wilted:

3 cups fresh spinach, cut into strips

Add spinach and onions to tofu mixture. Spoon into baked pie crust and press in with spoon so top is uniform. Bake uncovered for 30 minutes at 350° until top is golden. For shiny finish, brush top of pie with olive oil immediately after removing from oven.

Variation:

For a creative alternative to whole wheat crust, use filo dough (available frozen in most markets). Follow directions on package. Spread half of filo sheets and cover with filling, then cover with remaining filo sheets. You may need to adjust the amount of filling.

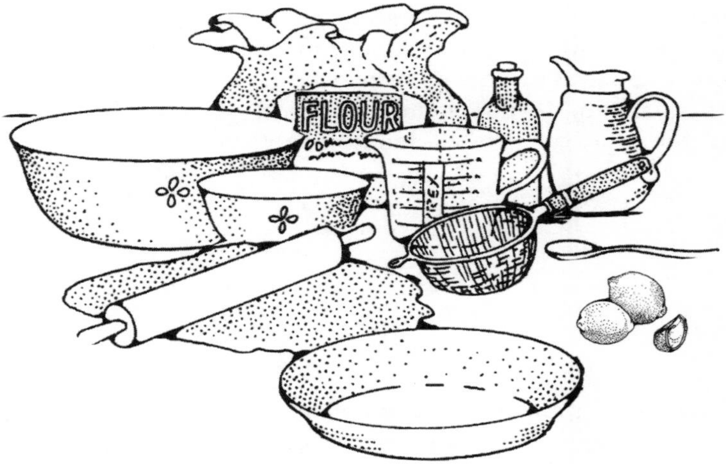

Maple Sesame Tofu

Surprisingly sweet and savory. A real crowd pleaser! Good served cold as a "to go" lunch.

Preparation time: 15 minutes
Marinating time: 20 – 60 minutes
Baking time: 20 minutes
Preheat oven to 350°

Serves: 4
Spring, Autumn, Winter

Mix in a bowl:

2 tablespoons maple syrup
3 tablespoons tamari or Bragg Liquid Aminos
2 tablespoons sunflower oil
1 tablespoon fresh ginger juice*
1 tablespoon sesame seeds

Drain:

1 pound firm tofu (not silken)

Slice each cube of tofu in half (lengthwise, so you have 2 squares the same size as the original, except half as thick). Cut each half into two triangles or rectangles, so each cube of tofu makes four pieces. Arrange tofu pieces on baking pan about 1" apart. Pour the mixture over the tofu slices. Allow to marinate for 20 – 60 minutes, turn pieces over and bake at 350° for approximately 20 minutes. Serve hot or cold.

**Grate ginger root, place small amount at a time into your palm, and squeeze juice into a bowl. Discard ginger pulp. You can also use a garlic press to squeeze fresh ginger: Place grated, unpeeled ginger in garlic press and squeeze juice into a bowl. ¼ teaspoon juice of ginger = 1 teaspoon grated ginger.*

Savory Tofu

Pleasing texture and taste with a smooth, gravy coating.

Preparation time: 20 minutes
Marinating time: Up to 1 hour
Baking time: 35 – 50 minutes
Preheat oven to 350°

Serves: 4 – 6
All Year

Slice into rectangles and brush with olive oil:

1½ pound firm tofu (not silken)—makes 12 pieces

Bake tofu on baking tray until golden at 350° (about 20 – 30 minutes).

Meanwhile, blend in a blender until smooth:

½ cup water
¼ cup tamari or Bragg Liquid Aminos
2" long ginger root, peeled and sliced
1 teaspoon dried basil
3 cloves garlic, peeled
2 teaspoons arrowroot powder

Pour the mixture on the baked tofu slices. Marinate for up to 1 hour (optional). Return to oven and bake at 350° for 10 minutes. Remove from oven, turn slices over, and bake for 5 – 10 more minutes. Serve hot or cold.

Vegetable Tofu Patties

Delicious and creative way to enjoy tofu—and a great substitute burger for hamburger lovers.

Preparation time: 35 minutes
Baking time: 20 – 30 minutes
Preheat oven to 350°

Serves 5: (8 – 10 patties)
All Year

Sauté until onions are golden brown:

2 tablespoons sunflower oil
1 medium onion, minced

Add and sauté for 5 minutes:

1 celery stalk, minced
1 medium carrot, peeled and grated

Add and sauté for 3 minutes:

1 teaspoon salt
1 teaspoon garlic powder
2 cups fresh spinach, minced

Set aside.

Meanwhile, blend in food processor until crumbled.

1½ pounds firm tofu (not silken)

Mix all ingredients together. Add to the mixture:

¼ cup sesame seeds, roasted

Form mixture into patties (see Appendix D, page 185). Bake on oiled baking tray at 350° for 20 – 30 minutes until golden. (A 10"x15" baking tray can hold 8 patties.)

Serving idea: serve with Mushroom Gravy.

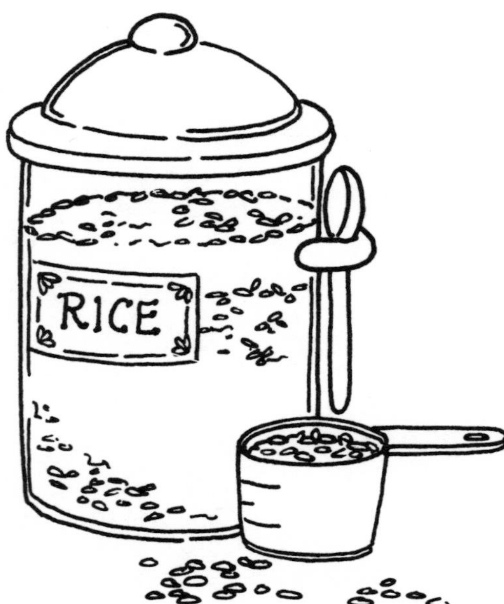
RICE

Grains

The Secret of Radiant Health and Well-Being is …

Proper diet; eating foods that are rich in vitality. If possible, eat in a harmonious environment, not in places where there is discord.

Introduction to Grains

Whole grains have wonderful grounding and calming qualities. They can be boiled, baked, pressure cooked, roasted, or fried. They can be cooked with water or, for a more flavorful taste, vegetable broth.

Before cooking grains, rinse them at least 3 times in cold water. Water should be relatively clear in the last rinsing.

Some grains take longer to cook than others. (For example, brown rice takes longer to cook and needs more water than white rice.) The amount of water needed and the time of cooking may vary with the amount of grain cooked, altitude, weather, temperature, etc. Once the grain is cooked thoroughly—once it's soft and has absorbed all the water—remove from heat and let stand covered for 5–10 minutes. This allows the steam within the pot to finish the process of cooking.

When cooking rice, bring to a boil, cover, and simmer. Do not stir the rice during this time. Our rice recipes use mainly white basmati rice—a light grain that is easy to digest for all body constitutions. In autumn and winter, you may wish to substitute brown rice for white basmati rice.

Roasting Grains, Nuts & Seeds

Grains

Dry roasting grains, especially short grain brown rice and millet, adds a nice aroma and flavor to the dish. Place grain in a dry skillet (no oil) in a single layer. Dry roast over medium heat for 2–10 minutes, stirring constantly. Roast grain until fragrant and lightly browned. (Whole grains will pop when done.) This gives grains a rich, nutty flavor.

Nuts and Seeds

Place one layer of any kind of seed or nut in a skillet. Dry roast (no oil) over low to medium heat until fragrant, beginning to pop, and getting lightly brown. Stir often or shake the skillet every 30 seconds for about 5–10 minutes (depending on the seeds or nuts). Remove from heat and let sit for a few minutes to complete the process of roasting.

For larger amounts you can use the oven. Place one layer of seeds or nuts on an ungreased baking tray. Place in a preheated oven at 350° for 10–30 minutes, depending on the seeds or nuts. Stir occasionally, roasting until fragrant, beginning to pop, and lightly brown.

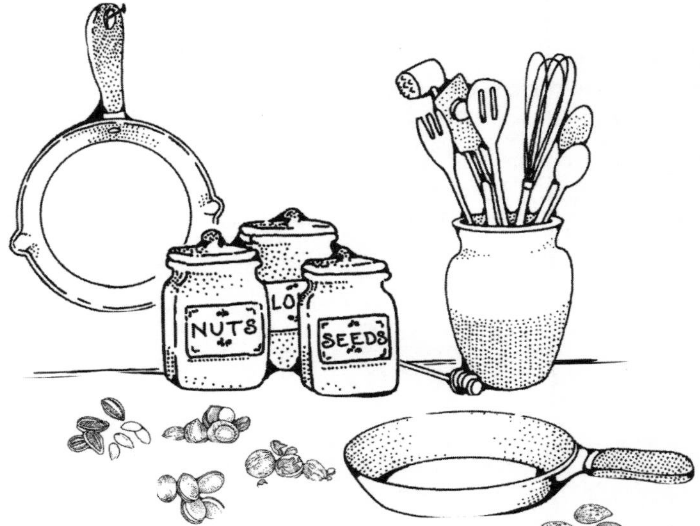

Plain Rice

Like everything else, cooking rice is easy—once you know how to do it.

Cooking time: 15 – 30 minutes

Serves: 3 – 4
All Year

For white rice: In a saucepan bring to a boil:

2 cups water
1 pinch salt

While water is coming to a boil, thoroughly rinse for several minutes:

1 cup white rice

Add rice to water, reduce heat, cover and simmer over low heat until all water is absorbed. Turn off heat and let stand, covered, for 10 minutes. Fluff with fork before serving.

For brown rice: In a saucepan bring to a boil:

2½ cups water
1 cup brown rice (rinsed several times)
1 pinch salt

Reduce heat, cover and simmer over low heat until all water is absorbed. Turn off heat and let stand, covered, for 10 minutes. Fluff with fork before serving.

Simple Tasty Rice

Cooking the rice with broth instead of water adds a special flavor.

Preparation time: 30 minutes
Cooking time: 30 minutes

Serves: 8
Spring, Summer

For the broth, put in a pot:

6 cups water
2 carrots, peeled and minced
4 stalks celery, minced

You can use a food processor to mince the carrots and celery. Bring to a boil and simmer for 10 minutes.

Add:

1 bunch fresh parsley, minced, with stems
1 cup fresh spinach, cut into strips

Simmer for 10 more minutes. Strain and keep the broth (discarding vegetables).

Sauté for 3–5 minutes:

2 tablespoons olive oil
4 green onions, cut into thin rounds
½ teaspoon black pepper

Mix the broth and sautéed green onions. Bring to a boil and add:

1 teaspoon salt
3 cups white basmati rice (rinsed 3 times)

Simmer until water is absorbed and rice is cooked. Turn heat off and let stand, covered, for 10 minutes. Fluff with a fork.

Summer Rice Salad

Easy to prepare, light, and colorful.

Preparation time: 20 minutes
Cooking time: 15 – 25 minutes

Serves: 6 – 8
Spring, Summer

Bring to a boil:

3 cups water
1 pinch salt

Add:

1½ cups white basmati rice (rinsed 3 times)

Bring to a boil and simmer until all water is absorbed and rice is cooked (approximately 10–15 minutes).

Meanwhile, sauté until onions are golden:

2 tablespoons sunflower oil
1 tablespoon olive oil
1 cup onions, minced

Add to onions:

2 green onions, minced
½ cup red bell pepper, cubed
1 medium zucchini, cut into quarter rounds
1 cup frozen corn, thawed

Sauté and stir together until vegetables are cooked but still crisp (add water if needed). Mix vegetables with rice and add:

¼ cup fresh parsley, minced
¼ cup fresh dill, minced
salt and black pepper to taste

Serve warm or cold.

Serving idea: Serve with Lemon Tomato Sauce or Vitality Dressing.

Rice with Red Bell Peppers

Creative, elegant-yet-simple rice dish.

Preparation time: 20 minutes
Cooking time: 10–15 minutes
Baking time: 5–10 minutes
Preheat oven to 350°

Serves: 6
All Year

Bring to a boil:
4 cups water

Add:
2 cups white basmati rice (rinsed 3 times)

Simmer until all water is absorbed and rice is cooked (approximately 10–15 minutes). Set aside.

Sauté for 3–5 minutes:
3 tablespoons olive oil
6 green onions, minced
¼ cup pine nuts
½ red bell pepper, cubed

Mix sautéed vegetables with cooked rice, adding salt and black pepper to taste. Ladle rice into oiled baking tray, so rice is arranged in small mounds. Bake at 350° for 5–10 minutes. Garnish with parsley.

Festive Rice

Tantalizing and naturally sweet.

Preparation time: 20 minutes
Cooking time: 10–15 minutes

Serves: 6–8
All Year

Sauté until onions are golden:

2 tablespoons olive oil
1 cup onions, minced

Set aside. Sauté in same pan for 3 minutes:

2 tablespoons olive oil
2 green onions, minced

Add to pan with green onions and sauté for 5 minutes:

3 tablespoons pine nuts
1 tomato, peeled then cut into cubes (put whole tomato in hot water for one minute, then peel skin)

Set aside.

Bring to a boil:

4 cups water
1 pinch allspice
¼ teaspoon cinnamon

Add to spiced boiling water:

2 cups white basmati rice (rinsed 3 times)

Simmer until water is absorbed and rice is cooked (approximately 10–15 minutes).

Mix in a serving bowl all ingredients and add:

1 teaspoon salt (or to taste)
¼ teaspoon black pepper (or to taste)

Serve warm.

Serving idea: For a festive presentation, fill a ladle with the mixture and flatten the top. Turn it with flat side on a plate and add a sprig of parsley to the top of the mound. For a special occasion, serve rice in baked acorn squash halves.

Baked Lemon Rice

Light and tangy. Great for a festive meal.

Preparation time: 25 minutes
Cooking time: 60 minutes
Preheat oven to 350°

Serves: 8
All Year

Bring 3 cups water to a boil, turn off heat and add:
2 tablespoons powdered vegetable broth

Set aside.

Sauté until onions are translucent:
2 tablespoons ghee, or sunflower oil
1 medium onion, minced

Place in an 8"x8" glass baking pan:
2 cups white basmati rice (rinsed 3 times)

Mix sautéed onions into rice. Then pour over rice and onions:
vegetable broth (prepared above)
3 tablespoons fresh lemon juice

Cover with foil and bake at 350° for 60 minutes (until all liquid is absorbed).

Remove from oven, open foil and sprinkle with:
2 tablespoons lemon peel
½ cup fresh chives, minced

Season with salt and pepper and stir until well combined.

Variation for vegetable broth.

Combine in pot:
5 cups cold water
1 unpeeled carrot, cut into big chunks
½ bunch fresh parsley, whole
2 celery stalks, cut into diagonals

Bring to a boil. Simmer for 15 minutes. Strain into a large bowl, saving the broth (discarding vegetables). Use 3 cups of broth instead of water and powdered vegetable broth.

Mexican Rice

A colorful, flavorful rice dish.

Preparation time: 20 minutes
Cooking time: 15–20 minutes

Serves: 6–8
Spring, Autumn

Place in a pot and bring to a boil:

5 cups water

Add:

2½ cups white basmati rice or jasmine rice (rinsed 3 times)

Simmer until water is absorbed and rice is cooked, approximately 10–15 minutes.

Meanwhile, sauté in pan 3–5 minutes:

¼ cup olive oil
1 red bell pepper, thinly sliced ¾" long
4 green onions, thinly sliced

Add:

1 tablespoon dried oregano
1 tablespoon chile powder
3 cloves garlic, peeled and minced
1 serrano chile, seeded and finely minced (optional)

Sauté for 3–5 minutes. Add:

2 tablespoons tomato paste
¼ cup water
1 cup frozen corn, thawed (optional)

Mix and cook for 3 minutes. Add cooked rice and sauté an additional 5 minutes. Add salt to taste.

Serving idea: Serve with Mexican Vegetables and tortillas.

Rice with Pasta

A tasty grain partnership with an appealing combination of colors—serve it with Pesto Vinaigrette.

Preparation time: 10 minutes
Cooking time: 10–15 minutes

Serves: 3–4
Spring, Summer

In a pot, melt:

3 tablespoons ghee or butter

Add:

½ cup spinach pasta (or sesame pasta) broken into pieces approximately ½" long

Stir and coat pasta with butter for 3–5 minutes. Add:

1 cup white basmati rice (rinsed 3 times)

Stir and coat rice for 2 minutes. Add:

3 cups water
½ teaspoon salt

Cook until all water is absorbed and rice is done (approximately 10–15 minutes).

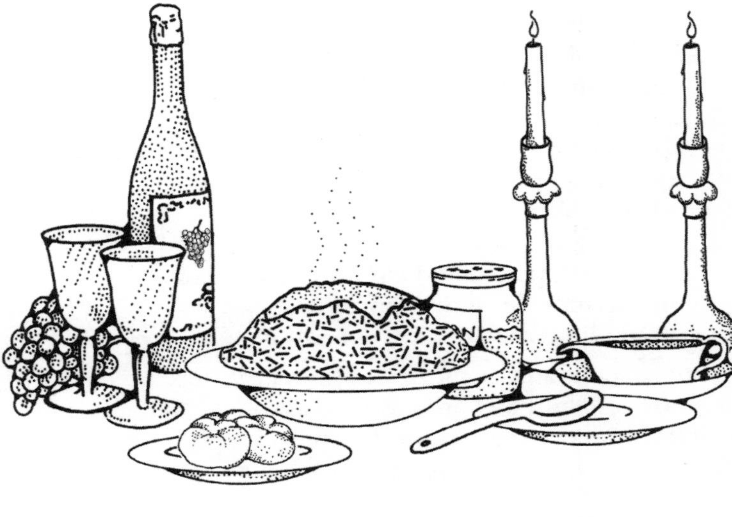

Kitchari

Nourishing and fulfilling. A simple Indian stew of rice, red lentils, vegetables, and spices. It is easy to digest and assimilate.

Preparation time: 30 minutes	Serves: 6
Cooking time: 30–40 minutes	Autumn, Winter

Bring to a boil then reduce heat and simmer for 15 minutes:

⅔ cup red lentils, washed and rinsed
3 cups water

Strain lentils and set aside.

Sauté in a pot:

2 tablespoons ghee or butter
3½ teaspoons mustard seeds
2 teaspoons cumin seeds

When mustard seeds start to pop, add:

1¼ teaspoons turmeric
2½ tablespoons fresh ginger, grated

Sauté about 5 minutes on low heat.

Add to the spices and mix:

cooked lentils
1½ cups white basmati rice (rinsed 3 times)
5 cups water or vegetable broth
½ cup green beans (fresh or frozen), cut into 1½" pieces
½ cup onions, minced
½ cup green cabbage, minced
½ cup celery, minced
½ cup carrots, peeled and cut into half rounds
½ cup zucchini, cut into rounds (or
½ cup butternut squash, cubed)

Bring to a boil and simmer on low heat (use a flame diffuser to avoid burning) until water is absorbed and rice and vegetables are cooked (approximately 15–20 minutes). Cook until beans and rice are very soft, but not gummy. Add water if needed to ensure rice is cooked completely.

After the kitchari is done, stir in:

2 teaspoons salt or tamari or Bragg Liquid Aminos, or to taste
black pepper (to taste)
⅓ cup fresh cilantro leaves

Serve with Date-Raisin Chutney or Apple Chutney.

Indian Herbed Rice

A blend of herbs that makes rice taste and smell wonderful.

Preparation time: 5 minutes
Cooking time: 35 minutes
Serves: 6–8
Autumn, Winter

Sauté in small pot until mustard seeds start to pop:

2 tablespoons ghee or sunflower oil
2 teaspoons brown mustard seeds
2 teaspoons cumin seeds

Stir in:

2 cups white basmati rice (rinsed 3 times)
3 tablespoons tamari or Bragg Liquid Aminos
2½ tablespoons dried basil
1½ tablespoons dried dill weed
1½ teaspoons powdered ginger
4 cups water

Bring to a boil, then lower heat, cover, and simmer until rice is cooked and all water is absorbed (approximately 30 minutes). Remove from heat and let stand, covered, for 5–10 minutes. Fluff with fork.

Serving idea: Serve with Vegetable Wraps, Sweet Tomato Sauce, Date-Raisin Chutney and Cilantro Beets.

Squash-Rice Combo

A nice, creamy variation on the traditional Italian risotto. Does not require oil or stirring.

Preparation time: 20 minutes — Serves: 6
Cooking time: 25 – 35 minutes — Autumn, Winter

Bring to a boil and simmer until rice is cooked (approximately 10–15 minutes):

1 cup brown basmati rice (rinsed 3 times)
2½ cups vegetable broth (2½ cups boiling water and 1 tablespoon powdered vegetable broth)*

In another pot, place ½ cup water with:

1 cup onions, minced

Simmer until onions are translucent.

Add:

1 cup water
3 cups butternut squash, peeled and cubed
1 teaspoon ground coriander
1 teaspoon dried parsley
1 teaspoon salt
¼ teaspoon nutmeg

Cook until squash is soft (approximately 15–20 minutes). You may need to add water. Mix cooked rice with squash. Add salt to taste.

** For fresh vegetable broth, see Baked Lemon Rice recipe, p. 113.*

Coconut Rice

A different and delicious way to enjoy rice.

Preparation time: 20 minutes
Cooking time: 15 – 20 minutes

Serves: 6
Autumn, Winter

Sauté in a large pot for 5 minutes:

1 – 2 tablespoons olive oil
1 – 2 tablespoons sunflower oil
2 small zucchini, cut into half rounds
1 carrot, peeled and cut into quarter rounds
1 cup fresh green beans (or frozen)
2 tablespoons grated ginger

Add and bring to a boil:

4 cups water

Stir in:

½ cup coconut, shredded
1½ teaspoons salt
2 cups white basmati rice (rinsed 3 times)

Boil again and reduce heat. Cover and simmer on low heat until all the water is absorbed (approximately 10 – 15 minutes). Turn heat off and let sit for 5 – 10 minutes before serving.

Serving idea: Good with our vegetable soups and Rye Bread.

Plain Millet

A light grain with a pleasing texture. An alternative to rice.

Cooking time: 15 – 25 minutes

Serves: 3 – 4
Spring, Summer, Autumn

In saucepan boil:

3 cups water
1 pinch salt

While water is coming to a boil, thoroughly rinse in a strainer for several minutes:

1 cup millet

Add millet to water, reduce heat, cover and simmer until all water is absorbed. Turn off heat. Let sit covered for 5 minutes. Fluff with fork.

Variation:

Dry roast the millet before adding to boiling water for a rich nutty flavor (make sure to wash millet first).

Serving ideas: Good with Tahini Sauce and Magic Vegetable Topping.

Cauliflower Millet

Gives body and a nice flavor to millet, especially when served with Tahini Sauce.

Preparation time: 10 minutes
Cooking time: 30 – 40 minutes

Serves: 6 – 8
All Year

Put in a pot and cook until all water is absorbed:

1½ cups millet (rinsed 2 – 3 times)
3 cups cauliflower florets, cut into small pieces
6 cups water
3 teaspoons dried basil
3 teaspoons dried thyme
3 teaspoons tamari or Bragg Liquid Aminos
1 teaspoons salt

Bring to a boil, cover and simmer (use flame diffuser if possible) for 30 – 40 minutes. Lightly stir cooked millet and season with salt to taste.

Plain Bulgur

A light whole wheat grain. Good substitute for rice, especially on a hot day.

Cooking time: 15 minutes

Serves: 3 – 4
Spring, Summer

Place in bowl:

1 cup bulgur
1½ cups boiling water

Cover and let sit for 10 minutes. Fluff with fork.

Serving ideas: Good with Sweet Zucchini Salad or Herbed Vegetables.

Bulgur Garbanzo Salad

A light yet satisfying main dish. A crowd pleaser.

Preparation time: 40 minutes
Soaking time: Overnight
Cooking beans: 60–90 minutes

Serves: 10
Spring, Summer

Soak overnight in 3 cups water:
1 cup garbanzo beans

Drain and rinse garbanzo beans. Place in a pot:
soaked garbanzo beans
water 3"–4" above level of beans

Bring to a boil, reduce heat to simmer and cook until soft (but not mushy) approximately 60–90 minutes. Meanwhile place in a bowl:
2½ cups bulgur

Pour over bulgur:
3½ cups boiling water

Cover and let sit for 10 minutes.

Add to bulgur and mix:
1 cup fresh parsley, minced
¼ cup fresh basil, sliced into thin strips
⅓ cup reconstituted sun dried tomatoes, minced (to reconstitute sun dried tomatoes, pour 1 cup boiling water over tomatoes and soak for 15 minutes, or until soft)
½ teaspoon dried oregano
1 teaspoon black pepper
1½ teaspoons salt (or to taste)
⅓ cup olive oil
⅓ cup fresh lemon juice

Serve immediately or cover and place in warm oven until ready to serve.

Variations:

1. Use short grain brown rice instead of bulgur and follow rice cooking procedure.

2. Instead of sun dried tomatoes, oregano, and basil, use ¼ cup minced fresh mint leaves and ½ cup green onions cut into thin rounds.

Barley Salad

Soothing and nourishing.

Preparation time: 20 minutes
Cooking time: 40 minutes

Serves: 8
Spring, Autumn, Winter

Rinse 2–3 times in cold water:
1½ cups barley

Add:
4 cups water

Bring to a boil and simmer until barley is soft and chewy (approximately 40 minutes).

Meanwhile, sauté for 5–8 minutes:
2 tablespoons sunflower oil
2 tablespoons olive oil
3 tablespoons sesame seeds
6–8 green onions, minced
3 cups mushrooms, sliced

Stir in and cook for 2 more minutes:
4 cups fresh spinach, cut into strips

Combine sautéed vegetables with cooked barley, along with:
3 tablespoons tamari or Bragg Liquid Aminos
¼ teaspoon black pepper

Serve warm.

Warm Couscous Salad

A festive, colorful, light salad.

Preparation time: 40 minutes

Serves: 8 – 10
Spring, Summer, Autumn

Place in a bowl:

2¼ cups boiling water
2¼ cups couscous or whole wheat couscous*

Cover and let sit for 10 minutes. Meanwhile mix together:

½ cup green or red bell pepper, diced
¼ cup red onion, diced
1 medium carrot, peeled and diced
½ cup quartered artichoke hearts
2 tablespoons capers (optional)
½ cup fresh parsley, minced
1 tablespoon fresh dill or 1 teaspoon dried dill weed
¼ cup raisins

Fluff couscous and add mixed vegetables. Cover and set aside. To make dressing, mix in a small bowl:

⅓ cup natural rice vinegar or white wine vinegar
½ cup olive oil
1 clove garlic, peeled and minced
1 teaspoon salt
1 teaspoon black pepper
½ teaspoon dried basil
½ teaspoon dried oregano
¼ cup fresh parsley, minced

Pour half of dressing over salad, taste. Add more as needed.

Variation:

Use short grain brown rice instead of couscous and follow rice cooking procedure.

* *Whole wheat couscous can be found in health food stores.*

Plain Quinoa

A nutritious complete protein. A light grain alternative to rice.

Cooking time: 15 – 25 minutes

Serves: 3 – 4
Spring, Summer, Autumn

In saucepan boil:

2 cups water
pinch salt

While water is coming to a boil, thoroughly rinse in a strainer for several minutes:

1 cup quinoa

Add quinoa to water, reduce heat, cover and simmer until all water is absorbed and quinoa becomes translucent and looks like partial spirals. Turn off heat. Let sit covered for 5 minutes. Fluff with fork.

Variation:

Dry roast the quinoa before adding to boiling water for a rich nutty flavor (make sure to wash quinoa first).

Serving ideas: Good with Tahini Sauce and Vegetable Empanada or topped with Lemon Ginger Dressing or Vitality Dressing.

Quinoa Salad

A light and nutritious salad. A feast for the eyes and the taste buds.

Preparation time: 20 minutes
Cooking time: 30 minutes

Serves: 6
Spring Summer Autumn

Bring to a boil:
2 cups water

Add:
1 cup quinoa (rinsed 3 times)
1 tablespoon powdered vegetable broth

Cover and simmer until all water is absorbed. Let sit covered for 5 minutes, then fluff.

While quinoa is cooking, sauté in a pan until golden:
2 tablespoons sunflower oil
1 tablespoon olive oil
1 cup onion or leek, minced

Add and sauté for 5 minutes:
1 cup red bell pepper
2 tablespoons poppy seeds

Mix cooked quinoa with sautéed vegetables and add:
1 green onion, minced
¾ cup carrot, peeled and grated
⅓ cup fresh parsley, minced
2 tablespoons fresh lemon juice
1 teaspoon Spike
½ teaspoon salt

Serve warm or cold.

Rice Patties

Satisfying and unusual way to enjoy rice. A winner!

Preparation time: 40 minutes
Cooking time: 10–15 minutes
Baking time: 15–20 minutes
Preheat oven to 350°

Serves: 5 (9–10 patties)
All Year

Bring to a boil and then simmer until all water is absorbed:

1 cup white, brown basmati, or sushi rice (rinsed 3 times)
3 cups water

Make sure rice is cooked and sticky. Set aside.

Sauté until onions are golden:

2 tablespoons sunflower oil
1 cup onions, minced
2 cloves garlic, peeled and minced

Add and sauté for 3 minutes:

1½ cups mushrooms, sliced

Set aside.

In a bowl, mix:

2 tablespoons fresh parsley, minced
1 teaspoon dried dill weed
1 teaspoon salt
¼ cup sunflower seeds, roasted

Add:

sautéed vegetables
cooked rice

Mix well and make into patties (see Appendix D, page 188). Place patties on oiled baking tray and bake at 350° for 15–20 minutes or until golden and crisp. (A 10"x15" baking tray can hold 8 patties.)

Serving idea: Serve with steamed vegetables and Tahini Sauce or Mushroom Gravy.

Millet Patties

Light yet satisfying. Great for snacking or lunch.

Preparation time: 45 minutes
Cooking time: 10–15 minutes
Baking time: 20–30 minutes
Preheat oven to 350°

Serves: 5 (8–10 patties)
All Year

Bring to a boil and simmer until all water is absorbed:

1 cup millet (rinsed 3 times)
4 cups water

Cover and set aside.

While millet is cooking, sauté until onions are golden brown:

2 tablespoons sunflower oil
1 cup onions, minced
1 clove garlic, peeled and minced

Add and sauté for 3 minutes:

1 cup carrots, peeled and grated

In a separate bowl, combine:

1 teaspoon salt
1 teaspoon dried dill weed
½ teaspoon dried thyme
¼ cup fresh parsley, minced
¼ cup sunflower seeds, roasted
½ cup bread crumbs or ½ cup cooked rice

Add cooked vegetables and millet to the bowl, and mix well.

Make patties (see Appendix D, page 188), place on oiled baking tray, and bake at 350° for 20–30 minutes. (A 10"x15" baking tray can hold 8 patties.)

Serving idea: Serve with steamed vegetables and Tahini Sauce or Mushroom Gravy.

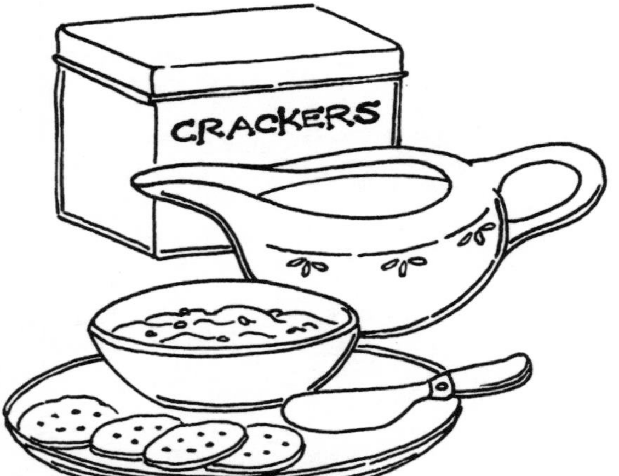
CRACKERS

Sauces and Spreads

The Secret of Radiant Health and Well-Being is . . .

Happiness within, radiated outward in a sense of well-being to others. Happiness is the fruit of faith in life, in God, in one's own high potential.

- Zucchini-Carrot Sauce
- Magic Vegetable Topping
- Apricot Dijon Sauce
- Tahini Sauce
- Miso Sauce
- Spinach-Mushroom Sauce
- Mushroom Gravy
- Golden Gravy
- Tomato Pizza Sauce
- Lemon Tomato Sauce
- Sweet Tomato Sauce
- Olive Spread
- Potato-Garlic Spread
- Pesto
- Pesto Vinaigrette
- Date-Raisin Chutney
- Apple Chutney
- Cucumber Raita
- Dipping Sauce
- Herbed Ghee

Zucchini-Carrot Sauce

Excellent alternative to regular gravy. Especially good on Plain Rice and Seasoned Spinach Salad.

Preparation time: 15 minutes
Cooking time: 15 – 20 minutes
Makes: 2 cups
Spring, Summer

Sauté in a small pot until onions are golden:

2 tablespoons olive oil
1 medium onion, minced

Add and sauté for 5 minutes, stirring frequently:

1 medium carrot, peeled and cut into quarter rounds
2 medium zucchini, cut into half rounds

Sprinkle to coat the vegetables:

3 tablespoons whole wheat pastry flour

Stir in:

¾ cup water

Cook on low heat, using a flame diffuser if possible, until vegetables are soft. Stir frequently to prevent burning. Blend in food processor until smooth. Add salt and pepper to taste.

Magic Vegetable Topping

Great over Plain Rice, mashed potatoes, and pasta.

Preparation time: 20 minutes
Cooking time: 10 minutes
Makes: 1½ cups
Spring, Summer

Sauté until onions are golden brown:

1 – 2 tablespoons sunflower oil
1 – 2 tablespoons olive oil
1 medium red onion, minced

Add and sauté for 5 minutes:

2 stalks celery, minced
1 medium carrot, peeled and minced

Add:

½ cup water

Cover and simmer for 10 minutes. Then add:

1 medium soft tomato, cubed
½ teaspoon salt
1 teaspoon dried oregano

Cover and simmer for 5 minutes longer. Serve immediately.

Variation:

Replace the celery with half a parsnip.

Apricot Dijon Sauce

A sweet and tangy combination.

Cooking time: 5 minutes

Serves: 6 – 8
All Year

Blend in a blender until smooth:

½ cup apricot jam
1 – 2 tablespoons Dijon mustard
½ cup water

Place in a sauce pan, heat gently and mix well.

Serving idea: Serve with Veggie Paté or Walnut Balls.

Tahini Sauce

Thick and hearty sauce—great on Stuffed Cabbage, Vegetable Pasties, and Patties (Rice, Millet, or Tofu).

Preparation time: 15 – 20 minutes
Cooking time: 5 minutes

Makes: 1 cup
Spring, Autumn, Winter

Sauté in a pot until onions are golden:

- **3 tablespoons sunflower oil**
- **1 small onion, minced**
- **2 tablespoons fresh ginger, peeled and grated**

Add:

- **⅓ cup raw tahini**
- **⅓ cup plus 2 tablespoons water**
- **2 tablespoons tamari or Bragg Liquid Aminos**
- **1 tablespoon maple syrup**
- **¼ teaspoon black pepper**

Stir with a wooden spoon and simmer for 5 minutes. Blend all ingredients in a food processor until smooth. Add salt to taste. Before serving, mix into the sauce:

- **¼ cup fresh parsley or fresh dill, minced**

Variation:

After blending all the ingredients in food processor, add ½ cup sliced mushrooms that have been sautéed in olive oil.

Miso Sauce

Grounding and soothing. Try it with Vegetable Empanada or cooked brown rice.

Preparation time: 15 minutes

Makes: 1¼ cups
All Year

Mix in a bowl:

2 tablespoons mellow miso
1½ cup warm vegetable broth (1½ cups boiling water and 1½ teaspoons powdered vegetable broth)

Dissolve the miso completely in the broth. Set aside.

Sauté in a small pot for 3–5 minutes:

2 tablespoons olive oil
6–8 green onions, minced (green and white parts)

Add:

½ cup garbanzo flour or barley flour (available at health food stores)

Add:

1 tablespoon tamari or Bragg Liquid Aminos
miso broth*

Mix well. Simmer for a few minutes. Gravy will be thick; you can add more water to dilute. If there are lumps, you can blend in a blender for a smoother consistency.

Variation:

In addition to green onions, you can also sauté ½ cup sliced mushrooms and add to gravy after it has been blended.

** Do not boil after adding miso, as that will cause the miso to lose its beneficial digestive enzymes.*

Spinach-Mushroom Sauce

Excellent on baked potatoes as a substitute for butter, sour cream, or traditional gravy.

Preparation time: 20 minutes

Makes: 2½ cups
All Year

Sauté until onions are translucent:

1–2 tablespoons sunflower oil
1–2 tablespoons olive oil
3 cups onions, minced

Add and sauté for 5 minutes:

1 cup mushrooms, sliced

Sprinkle and mix well:

¼ cup garbanzo flour (available at health food stores)

Add:

2 tablespoons fresh lemon juice
2 tablespoons tamari or Bragg Liquid Aminos
1 cup frozen chopped spinach, thawed and drained
1½ cups water

Mix thoroughly until it becomes a smooth sauce. Serve warm.

Mushroom Gravy

Great with Vegetable Pasties, Tofu Puff Pasties, and Patties (Rice, Millet, or Tofu).

Preparation time: 20 minutes

Makes: 1¼ cups
All Year

Sauté for 5 minutes:

2–4 tablespoons olive oil
1½ cups mushrooms, sliced

Mix in a small pot and simmer:

1 cup vegetable broth (1 cup boiled water and 1½ teaspoons powdered vegetable broth)
3 tablespoons tamari or Bragg Liquid Aminos
fresh ginger juice* (2" piece)

Add the sautéed mushrooms to simmering mixture.

Mix in a bowl:

2 tablespoons cold water
1 tablespoon arrowroot powder

Add to the mushroom mixture and stir frequently until liquid thickens.

** Grate ginger root, place small amount at a time into your palm, and squeeze juice into a bowl. Discard ginger pulp. You can also use a garlic press to squeeze fresh ginger: Place grated, unpeeled ginger in garlic press and squeeze juice into a bowl.*

Golden Gravy

A good substitute for chicken or turkey gravy—smooth and silky.

Cooking time: 20 minutes

Makes: 2 cups
Autumn, Winter

In a sauce pan, toast until lightly brown (approximately 5–7 minutes), making sure not to burn:

¼ cup nutritional yeast
¼ cup garbanzo, unbleached white, or whole wheat flour

Add and cook for 5 minutes, stirring frequently:

3 tablespoons sesame oil
3 tablespoons olive oil

Whisk in:

2 cups vegetable stock or hot water

Add:

1 tablespoon Dijon mustard
¼ cup tamari
1 large clove garlic, peeled and minced
1 teaspoon balsamic vinegar
½ teaspoon black pepper (or to taste)

Simmer 5–10 minutes, stirring frequently.

Serving idea: Good with Vegetable Paté or Vegetable Pasties.

Tomato Pizza Sauce

A nice blend of herbs that makes for an extraordinary pizza.

Preparation time: 10 minutes
Cooking time: 10 minutes

Makes: 2½ cups
All Year

Mix in a sauce pan:

1½ cups tomato purée (canned; avoid tomato paste, as it is too thick)
1½ cups water
1½ tablespoons dried basil
1½ tablespoons dried parsley
1½ tablespoons dried oregano
1½ tablespoons olive oil
2¼ teaspoons garlic powder
2¼ teaspoons onion powder
2¼ teaspoons salt
¼ teaspoon dried marjoram
¼ teaspoon dried thyme

Simmer for 10 minutes. Stir in:

1½ tablespoons honey

Use the Basic Whole Wheat Bread recipe for the crust of the pizza.

Lemon Tomato Sauce

Tangy tomato sauce. Great with Stuffed Cabbage.

Preparation time: 15 minutes
Cooking time: 5 minutes

Makes: 1¼ cups
All Year

Sauté until onions are translucent or slightly golden:

2 tablespoons sunflower oil
½ cup onions, minced

Add:

1½ cups ripe, soft tomatoes, minced

Mix tomatoes and sautéed onion, coating the tomatoes completely with onions. Add:

¼ cup apple juice
1 tablespoon fresh lemon juice

Simmer for 5 minutes. Place in a blender and blend until smooth. Pour into serving container and add salt and black pepper to taste (start with ½ teaspoon salt and a pinch of black pepper).

Sweet Tomato Sauce

Sweet and delicious. Good on Stuffed Cabbage, grains, and vegetables.

Preparation time: 15 minutes
Cooking time: 5 – 10 minutes

Makes: 1¾ cups
All Year

Sauté until onions are golden:

2 tablespoons sunflower oil
½ cup onions, minced

Add:

1½ cups soft, ripe tomatoes, minced

Stir together so that tomatoes are coated with onions. Add:

½ cup water

Bring to a boil and add:

1 teaspoon powdered vegetable broth
1 tablespoon fresh lemon juice
1 tablespoon maple syrup

Simmer for 5 minutes. Blend in a blender until smooth. Add salt and black pepper to taste.

Olive Spread

Excellent on Focaccia with tomato slices or red bell peppers. Also good with Whole Wheat Biscuits and French bread.

Preparation time: 10 minutes

Makes: 2 cups
All Year

Put in a food processor:

3 cups black olives, sliced (canned)
1 tablespoon dried oregano
1 large clove garlic, peeled and minced
⅓ cup olive oil

Blend using a pulse method so it has a coarse texture—be careful not to over-blend.

Potato-Garlic Spread

Great butter substitute. Delicious on Basic Whole Wheat Bread, Whole Wheat Sesame Crackers.

Preparation time: 20 minutes
Cooking time: 30 minutes
Preheat oven to 400°

Makes: 3 cups
All Year

Roast:

1 garlic bulb (**whole and not peeled**)

Wrap garlic in foil and roast at 400° for approximately 30 minutes until soft. Remove from oven and let cool.

Meanwhile, boil until soft:

3 russet potatoes, peeled and cubed

Strain and save water from cooking. Let potatoes cool for 5 minutes.

Place in a food processor and blend until smooth:

boiled potatoes
1 tablespoon dried chives (optional)
3 tablespoons olive oil
2 tablespoons fresh lemon juice
1 teaspoon salt

Take garlic out of foil and squeeze garlic into mixture in food processor. (It will be like a paste.) Blend together until smooth. Add a small amount of cooking water if you prefer a thinner consistency.

Pesto

Great with pasta or as a substitute for Tomato Pizza Sauce.

Preparation time: 10 minutes

Makes: 1 cup
All Year

Put in a food processor and blend until smooth:

2 cups fresh spinach
3 tablespoons dried basil
2 cloves garlic, peeled
2 tablespoons almonds or sunflower seeds
½ cup olive oil

Place blended mixture in a bowl and fold in:

3 tablespoons of mellow miso or
½ cup Parmesan cheese

Serve with pasta of your choice. Cook pasta until desired texture. Use 2 ounces of pasta per person and 2 tablespoons of pesto per person. Coat pasta with pesto after draining, while pasta is still warm, or you can serve the pesto on the side. Also great on pizza as a substitute for traditional tomato sauce.

Variation:

Instead of spinach and dried basil, you can use:

1 cup fresh spinach
1 cup fresh basil leaves (remove stems)

Pesto Vinaigrette

Distinctive flavor and an appealing green color. Serve on Plain Rice with Pasta or steamed vegetables.

Preparation time: 15 minutes — Makes: 1¼ cups
Spring, Summer

Blend in a blender or food processor:

1 cup packed fresh parsley leaves (remove stems)
1 cup packed fresh basil leaves
3 tablespoons fresh lemon juice
¾ cup olive oil
2 teaspoons prepared Dijon mustard

Blend until smooth.

Add:

½ teaspoon salt (or to taste)
1 pinch black pepper (or to taste)

Date-Raisin Chutney

A nice relish served as an accent to Kitchari or Indian food in general.

Preparation time: 15 minutes — Makes: 3 cups
Cooking time: 10–15 minutes — All Year

Place in a pot:

1 cup date pieces (or pitted fresh dates, cut into small pieces)
2 cups water, apple juice, orange juice or grape juice

Bring to a boil and simmer on low heat until dates are soft (approximately 5–10 minutes). Stir continuously and use a flame diffuser (if possible), as dates can burn easily.

Add:

2½ cups raisins
¼ teaspoon powdered ginger
¼ teaspoon nutmeg
¼ teaspoon ground cloves
¼ teaspoon cinnamon
½ teaspoon salt
1 pinch cayenne

Mix well and simmer for 5 minutes. Place in a food processor and blend until smooth.

Apple Chutney

A nice relish served as an accent to Kitchari or Indian food in general.

Preparation time: 15 minutes
Cooking time: 10–15 minutes
Makes: 2 cups
Autumn, Winter

Place in a pot:

1½ pounds green or red apples, peeled and sliced (about 3 apples)
1 tablespoon fresh ginger, peeled and grated
½ cup orange juice
1 teaspoon cinnamon
½ teaspoon ground cloves
1 teaspoon salt
½ cup water
1 pinch cayenne

Bring to a boil and simmer until apples are soft (approximately 10–15 minutes). Add:

¼ cup honey

Let cool for 5 minutes. Blend in a food processor until smooth. Serve warm or cold.

Cucumber Raita

Plain yogurt mixed with fresh grated vegetables and spices. It is served as a cooling complement to more spicy Indian dishes.

Preparation time: 10 minutes
Chilling time: 1 hour

Serves: 4
All Year

Mix together:

1 cup plain yogurt
1 cucumber, peeled seeded, grated and liquid squeezed out
1 tablespoon chopped fresh cilantro
½ teaspoon salt
½ teaspoon powdered cumin
⅛ teaspoon cinnamon

Chill for 1 hour or more.

Serving idea: Serve with Vegetable Garbanzo Curry or Moroccan Stew.

Dipping Sauce

A light, salty sauce that's great with Nori Rolls.

Cooking time: 5 minutes

Place in a small pot:

¼ cup water
¼ cup tamari or Bragg Liquid Aminos
1" piece of fresh ginger, sliced thin

Simmer at low heat for 5 minutes. Strain before serving. Add 1–2 teaspoons honey for less salty flavor.

Herbed Ghee

Fresh and light sauce with a nice lemony taste. Especially good on steamed broccoli or artichokes.

Preparation time: 10 minutes
Marinating time: 30 minutes

Makes: 1 cup
Spring, Summer

Melt:

¾ cup ghee or butter

Add to ghee and whisk together:

juice from 1 fresh lemon
½ teaspoon dried thyme
¼ teaspoon dried sage
¼ teaspoon salt (or to taste)

If possible, let sit for 30 minutes before serving or pouring on fresh vegetables. This allows flavors to blend more fully.

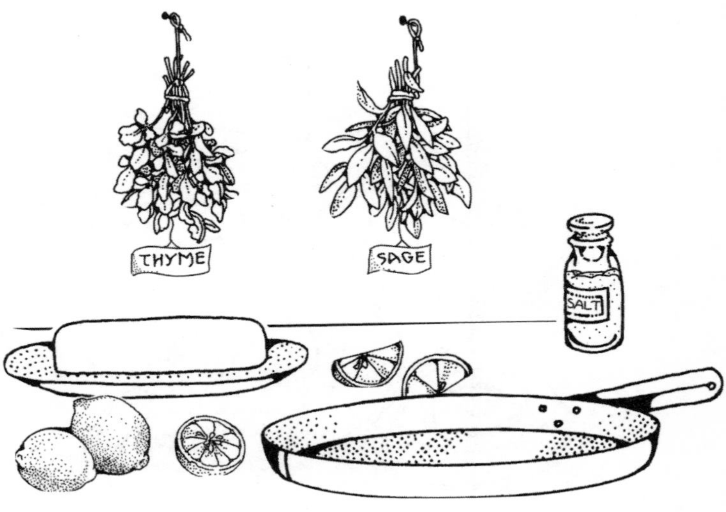

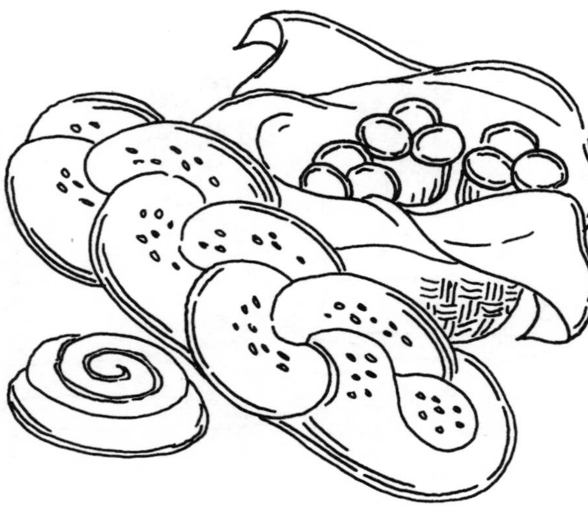

Breads

The Secret of Radiant Health and Well-Being is ...

Daily meditation. From the center of stillness within you, radiance will illuminate your entire being.

Pumpkin Bread

Great for breakfast or an afternoon snack—it's not too sweet.

Preparation time: 20 minutes
Baking time: 30 – 45 minutes
Preheat oven to 350°

Makes: 1 loaf (9"x5")
Autumn, Winter

Mix in a large bowl:

1 cup pumpkin (canned)
¼ cup sunflower oil
½ cup honey or maple syrup
1 teaspoon vanilla

Mix in a separate bowl:

½ teaspoon salt
1 teaspoon baking soda
½ teaspoon nutmeg
1 teaspoon cinnamon
1¾ cups whole wheat pastry flour

Mix dry ingredients into the wet ones. Fold until just mixed (do not over-mix). Spoon and spread into oiled 9" x 5" loaf pan and bake at 350° for 40–50 minutes or until center is set and toothpick inserted into center comes out clean. Cover with aluminum foil if top starts to brown too quickly.

Note: This bread keeps well if you wrap it in foil after it cools and freeze it.

Variation:

Replace pumpkin with 1 cup mashed ripe bananas.

Poppy Seed Cornbread

A moist, egg-less bread that goes well with soups and vegetables.

Preparation time: 20 minutes
Baking time: 40 – 60 minutes

Serves: 6 – 8
All Year

Thaw:
1 cup of frozen corn

Mix in a bowl:
1½ cups unbleached white flour
1 cup corn meal
½ teaspoon salt
1 tablespoon baking powder

Set aside.

In a bowl mix:
thawed corn
½ cup sunflower oil
1 cup water or rice milk

Mix dry ingredients into corn mixture.

Add:
1 tablespoon poppy seeds

Grease bottom and sides of an 8" x 8" glass baking pan. Spoon batter into pan and spread evenly. Bake at 350° for 40 – 60 minutes, or until toothpick inserted into center comes out clean.

Zucchini Breakfast Bread

Aromatic, delicious nonfat breakfast bread that's also perfect for afternoon tea. Great opportunity to use over-sized zucchini—especially fresh ones from your garden.

Preparation time: 25 minutes
Baking time: 50 – 60 minutes
Preheat oven to 350°

Makes: 1 loaf (9" x 5")
All Year

Mix in large bowl:

1 cup brown sugar
2 cups grated zucchini (with or without peel)
1 tablespoon vanilla extract
⅔ cup fresh orange juice
¾ cup raisins

In another bowl, mix:

1½ cups unbleached white flour
¾ cup whole wheat flour
1 teaspoon baking soda
1 teaspoon baking powder
1½ teaspoons cinnamon
¼ teaspoon allspice
¼ teaspoon ground cloves
1 teaspoon salt

Mix dry ingredients into wet ingredients until just blended. Spoon and spread into oiled 9" x 5" loaf pan. Bake at 350° for 50 – 60 minutes or until toothpick inserted into center comes out clean. Cover top with foil if it starts to brown too quickly (to keep it from burning).

Zucchini Dessert Bread

Sweet and satisfying dessert or afternoon snack.

Preparation time: 30 minutes
Baking time: 45 minutes
Preheat oven to 350°

Makes: 1 loaf (9" x 5")
All Year

Mix and set aside:

1 cup unbleached white flour
1 teaspoon baking powder
½ teaspoon baking soda
½ teaspoon cinnamon
¼ teaspoon nutmeg
⅛ teaspoon ground cloves
¼ teaspoon powdered ginger
¼ teaspoon salt

In a large bowl, mix:

⅓ cup sunflower oil
2 tablespoons fresh orange juice
½ cup maple syrup (use ¾ cup for a sweet tooth)
1 egg
1 cup zucchini (with or without peel), grated
⅓ cup raisins or unsweetened, shredded coconut
3 tablespoons walnuts, chopped

Mix dry ingredients into wet ones. Pour into oiled 9" x 5" loaf pan. Bake at 350° for 40–45 minutes or until toothpick inserted into center comes out clean. Cover top with foil if it starts to brown too quickly (to keep it from burning).

Serving idea: Very nice with your favorite whipped topping.

Barley Bread

A quick, nonfat, crusty country loaf.

Preparation time: 15 minutes
Baking time: 25 – 35 minutes
Preheat oven to 375°

Makes: 2 loaves
Autumn, Winter

Mix in a bowl:

1½ cups whole wheat flour
1 cup unbleached white flour
1 cup barley flour
1 teaspoon salt
1 teaspoon baking soda
1 teaspoon baking powder
2 tablespoon sesame seeds (optional)

Add and mix:

2 cups buttermilk or 2½ cups plain yogurt

The dough should be soft. With wet hands place dough on oiled baking tray. Form into 2 "baguette" shaped loaves. Using sharp knife, lightly make diagonal slits on surface of loaves. Bake 25 – 35 minutes at 375° until golden brown. Cool completely, then slice thin.

Whole Wheat Biscuits

A quick bread substitute to serve with your favorite soup or spread.

Preparation time: 20 minutes
Baking time: 12–15 minutes
Preheat oven to 400°

Makes: 12–13 biscuits
All Year

Mix in a large bowl:

2 cups whole wheat pastry flour
2 teaspoons baking powder
¼ teaspoon baking soda
½ teaspoon salt
1 teaspoon dried dill weed or Spike or Italian seasoning or 1 tablespoon fresh dill or thyme (optional)

Add:

¼ cup chilled butter (cut into small cubes)

Mix in butter (or use a pastry cutter) until the mixture has the consistency of coarse crumbs.

Add:

¾ cup plain or vanilla soy milk
2 teaspoons fresh lemon juice

Mix until the dough holds together. On a well floured surface, knead dough gently, just until dough is not sticky (approximately 1 minute). Roll dough lightly to ⅓" thickness. Cut with a biscuit cutter (2½" diameter). Place biscuits on an oiled baking sheet and bake at 400° for 12–15 minutes. Best served warm.

Variation

Substitute ¾ cup buttermilk or plain yogurt for soy milk and lemon juice.

Whole Wheat Sesame Crackers

It's easy to make your own healthy crackers—an excellent snack food.

Preparation time: 25 minutes
Baking time: 12–15 minutes
Preheat oven to 400°

Makes: 32 crackers
(3 x 1¼-inch)
Spring, Summer

Mix in a large bowl:

1¼ cups whole wheat flour
1 cup unbleached white flour
1 cup sesame seeds
1 teaspoon salt
1 cup water
3 tablespoons sunflower oil
2 teaspoons tamari or Bragg Liquid Aminos

Combine all ingredients until a dough is created. Knead for 2–3 minutes. Divide dough in two parts and place each half on an oiled baking sheet (11½" x 16½"). Roll and press dough from the center to all sides. Make sure to form an even surface. (Roll with even pressure out to the edges so that you get an even thickness throughout the tray. If dough is not a consistent thickness, the edges will burn while the center remains uncooked.) Cut dough into 3 x 4¼-inch rectangles. Each tray will make 16 crackers. Sprinkle lightly with salt (optional). Bake at 400° for 12–15 minutes or until golden-brown. Store in airtight container and use as a snack for the next few days.

Yeasted Breads

Here are basic techniques to use for the yeasted bread recipes that follow.

Preparing the Yeast Mixture

- Measure the water called for by the recipe into a small bowl (lukewarm—it should not feel warmer than your wrist, or else it might kill the active dry yeast, and the bread will not rise).
- Add the active dry yeast and stir lightly to dissolve.
- Add sweetener.
- Let stand until foamy, about 10 minutes.

Preparing the Dough

- Mix other ingredients according to recipe. Fold active dry yeast mixture into other ingredients in a bowl. Stir until dough holds together—dough will become thick and moist.
- Transfer the lump of dough to a clean, floured surface. Begin kneading until smooth and elastic.

Kneading the Dough

- *If kneading by mixer:* Use a mixer with a dough hook attachment, and let the dough knead for 10 minutes on low speed.
- *If kneading by hand:* Fold the dough in toward you (bringing the far edge in toward you). Push down and forward, using the heels of the hands. Then turn the dough ¼ turn. Repeat the folding movement. Turn the dough ¼ turn again (the turn is always in the same direction). Continue to turn, fold, and push for about 10 minutes, until the dough is smooth, uniform, and non-sticky—add flour if necessary.

The Rising Process

- Place the dough in an oiled bowl and turn it over, so the surface of the dough is oily (to prevent dryness). Cover the bowl with a damp towel and put in a warm place to rise. (It can take 30–90 minutes to rise, depending on the recipe). The dough has risen when it has doubled its bulk. The time for rising will vary with the altitude, weather conditions, and temperature.
- Take off the towel and "punch" down the dough (by pushing your fist steadily and firmly into dough) 25–30 times all over the dough. You can coat your fist with flour to prevent sticking.
- Cut into even pieces according to recipe. Knead each piece 5–6 times and shape.
- *If using a baking tray:* Oil the tray and place the shaped loaf on the tray. If baking more than one loaf on a tray, leave a 3–4" space between loaves. When baking rolls, leave a 1½–2" space between rolls.
- *If using a bread pan:* Oil the pan and place the dough into the pan. Press the dough hard into the corners and floor of the pan. Take the dough out again and return it upside down to the pan. This gives the bread a smooth-looking surface.
- Cover with a damp towel and let rise again (about 20 minutes).

Shaping the Bread: See Appendix B (page 183)

Baking the Bread

- Brush surface (see page 159).
- Cut the top with ½" deep slits to allow steam to escape (except in the case of rolls, where slits are not needed).
- Sprinkle with seeds or herbs according to recipe.
- Bake in preheated oven at 350°.
- Remove from oven when the bread is done. To check

whether the bread is done, check the color (according to the recipe and the type of surface brushing). Also, the bread should resound with a deep, hollow thump when tapped with finger on the bottom of the loaf (turn loaf upside down).

Cooling and Storing the Bread

- Remove from the pan or baking tray and let cool—ideally for 1 hour—before cutting and serving. Rolls can be served immediately after being taken out of the oven.
- After the bread is completely cooled, it may be kept in a sealed plastic bag in the refrigerator, or frozen (wrapped with foil) for later use.

Brushing the Surface of Yeasted Breads and Rolls

There are four basic ways to coat the surface of yeasted breads and rolls:

- **Egg-wash:** one egg beaten with 2 tablespoons water (brush before baking). Gives a golden-brown, shiny surface.
- **Milk:** brush before baking. Gives a brown-colored surface.
- **Ghee or Butter:** melt and brush before and after baking. Gives a soft surface.
- **Water:** sprayed during baking gives a crisp, French bread-type crust.

Always glaze dough **before** making cuts, slashes, or slits in bread.

Basic Whole Wheat Bread

This recipe forms the foundation for several other breads in this book, and it's wonderful by itself, too—especially when you eat it fresh and warm.

Preparation time: 30 minutes
Rising time: 50 minutes
Baking time: 20 – 40 minutes
Preheat oven to 350°

Makes: 1 loaf
All Year

Mix in a small bowl and let foam:

2 cups warm water
1½ teaspoons active dry yeast
1 teaspoon honey

Mix in large bowl:

3 cups whole wheat flour
2 cups unbleached white flour
1½ teaspoons salt
3 tablespoons sunflower, or olive oil

Fold foamed, active dry yeast mixture into flour mixture and mix thoroughly to create a dough. Place on floured surface and knead for 10 minutes. Oil a large bowl. Form dough into a ball and place it in an oiled bowl, turning the dough to coat it with oil. Cover bowl with a damp towel or plastic wrap. Let rise in a warm place (but not too warm) for 30 minutes or until dough has doubled in size. Then punch down and knead again for 2 minutes.

Shape the bread. (See Appendix B, page 183, for shaping illustrations—this bread can also be braided, made round, or made into rolls.) Place on an oiled 10" x 15" baking tray. Cover again and let rise for no more than 20 minutes (not longer, or else the dough will lose its elasticity).

Brush with egg-wash and bake at 350° for 20–40 minutes or until bread is golden brown. Let cool for 10–20 minutes before slicing.

Variation for 2 loaves:

Mix and let foam:

3½ cups warm water
1 tablespoon active dry yeast
2 teaspoons honey

Mix in large bowl:

6 cups whole wheat flour
4 cups unbleached white flour
1 tablespoon salt
6 tablespoons sunflower, or olive oil

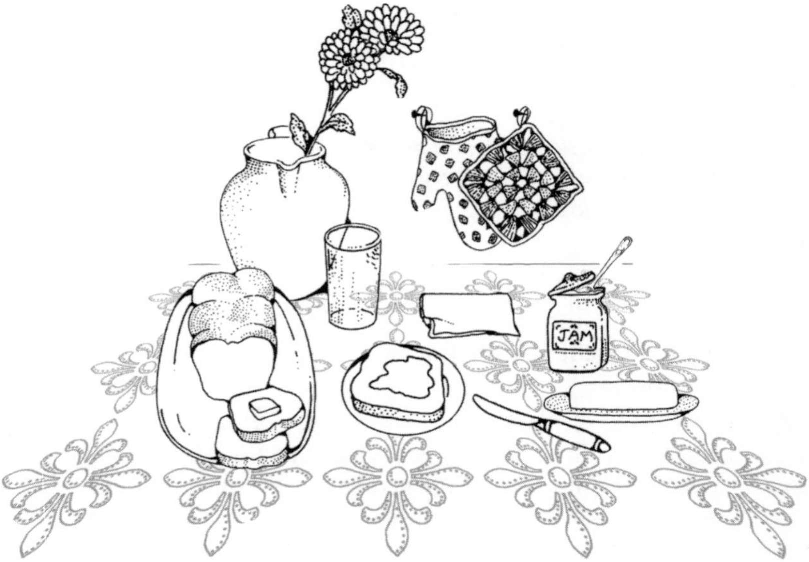

Carrot Pillows

Light as clouds and soft as pillows—they're not like any other dinner roll you've tasted. Bet you can't eat just one!

Preparation time: 45 minutes
Rising time: 1 hour
Baking time: 10–15 minutes
Preheat oven to 350°

Makes: 16-22 pillows
All Year

Boil until carrots are soft:

3 cups water
1½ medium carrots, peeled and cut into chunks

Drain and save water. Let carrots cool to room temperature for 10 minutes, then blend them in a blender or mash by hand.

While carrots are cooking, mix in a small bowl:

½ cup lukewarm water
1 tablespoon active dry yeast
1 teaspoon honey

Let foam for 5–10 minutes. Mix in a large bowl:

4 tablespoons olive oil
1 cup cooked and mashed carrots
2 tablespoons water from cooked carrots (or plain water)
1 tablespoon honey

Add foamed, active dry yeast mixture to carrot mixture. Combine ingredients thoroughly.

Mix in a separate bowl:

3 cups unbleached white flour
1 teaspoon salt

Add to carrot-yeast mixture and combine. Add more flour if needed. Place on floured surface and knead for 10 minutes and let rise for 40 minutes. Punch down and roll the dough to ¼" thickness. Cut into approximately 3" triangles (see illustration, Appendix B, page 186) and place on an oiled baking tray. Let rise for 20 minutes or until doubled in size.

Brush with egg-wash and bake at 350° for 10–15 minutes, or until golden. (You can sprinkle sesame seeds, poppy seeds, or dried dill weed on top of the egg-wash before baking.)

Variations:

Replace carrots with yams, winter squash, or potatoes.

Sesame Sticks

Soft, light, golden, melt-in-your-mouth bread sticks. Yum!

Preparation time: 30 minutes
Rising time: 35 minutes
Baking time: 10 minutes
Preheat oven to 350°

Makes: 8–10 sticks
Spring, Summer

Follow all instructions for Basic Whole Wheat Bread recipe for 1 loaf until dough has risen the first time. Then:

After dough has risen for the first time and been punched down, divide into 8–10 pieces. Cover with a towel.

In a large, shallow bowl, dissolve:

2 tablespoons baking soda
2 cups cold water

In another flat pan, spread ½ cup sesame seeds. Roll each piece of dough into a rope shape about 6"–8" long. Dip into baking soda solution, drain briefly on a kitchen towel and roll in sesame seeds (add more sesame seeds if needed). Place on an oiled baking tray, leaving 1½" between sticks. Let rise 5 minutes. Bake at 350° for 10 minutes or until golden brown. Cool briefly before serving.

Variation:

You can use a twist or figure "8" shape instead of a rope shape. (See Appendix B, page 183, for shaping illustrations.)

Spinach-Stuffed Bread

This substantial bread is almost a main dish. Add soup and salad for a complete, satisfying meal.

Preparation time: 45 minutes
Rising time: 40 minutes
Baking time: 20 – 30 minutes
Preheat oven to 350°

Makes: 2 rolled loaves
All Year

Follow directions for Basic Whole Wheat Bread for 1 loaf. While waiting for dough to rise for the first time, prepare filling for bread:

Sauté until onions are golden:

2 tablespoons sunflower oil
2 medium onions, cut into crescents
4 cloves garlic, peeled and minced

Add:

1 cup frozen spinach, thawed, squeezed dry, and firmly packed

Combine thoroughly, stirring for 5 minutes. Set aside.

In a separate bowl, crumble:

1 pound firm tofu (not silken)

Add:

¼ cup fresh lemon juice
¼ cup olive oil

Add spinach mixture to tofu mixture and combine all together. Add:

1½ teaspoons salt
1 teaspoon black pepper

Punch down dough and cut in half. Roll each half into a rectangle shape (8" x 15"). Spread half of the filling on each rectangle (leave 2" space on the 8" sides). Moisten the far-side 2" strip with water, roll starting from the near side, and adhere to the far side tightly. Place on oiled baking tray. Let rise for 10 minutes.

Brush surface of dough with egg-wash. Bake at 350° for 20–30 minutes or until light brown. Let cool and slice into 2" slices. Serve warm.

Rosemary Olive Bread

Aromatic and flavorful. Great with Hummus or Navy Bean Spread.

Preparation time: 30 minutes
Rising time: 50–55 minutes
Baking time: 30–35 minutes
Preheat oven to 350°

Makes: 2 small loaves
Spring, Autumn

Combine in a small bowl:

1 tablespoon active dry yeast
2 cups warm water
1 teaspoon honey

Let foam for 10 minutes.

In a separate bowl combine:

2 tablespoons olive oil
1 cup whole wheat flour
¼ cup fresh rosemary, minced, or 2 tablespoons dried rosemary
1 tablespoon salt
½ cup sliced black olives
4½ cups unbleached white flour

Add foamed, active dry yeast mixture to flour mixture. Mix well. Place on floured surface and knead for 10 minutes. Let rise for 30 minutes (or until doubled in size) and punch down. Shape into 2 round loaves and place on oiled baking tray. Let rise 20–25 minutes. Brush with egg-wash and bake at 350° for 30–35 minutes, or until golden brown.

Cinnamon Rolls

A simpler and healthier version of a traditional favorite—and with all the traditional flavor.

Preparation time: 45 minutes
Rising time: 50 minutes
Baking time: 15 – 20 minutes
Preheat oven to 350°

Makes: about 2 dozen
All Year

Use the Basic Whole Wheat Bread recipe for 1 loaf.

As the dough sits to rise for the first time, melt:

⅓ cup butter

Remove from heat and stir in:

⅔ cup honey

Set aside the honey-butter sauce. Mix in a separate bowl:

½ cup walnuts, chopped
1 cup raisins
1 tablespoon cinnamon

After dough has risen, punch down and turn out onto floured surface. Knead for 2 minutes and divide dough in half. Roll each half into a rectangle shape (10" x 14", and ⅜" thick—see illustrations, Appendix B, page 183).

Brush the surface lavishly with honey-butter sauce leaving a 2" space along each edge. Then sprinkle evenly with half of the walnut-raisin mixture. Moisten the far side strip with water, roll and adhere to the far side. Do the other half of the dough the same way.

Slice each roll into 12 pieces and place slices with spiral facing up on an oiled baking tray 2" apart. Cover with plastic wrap and let rise for 20 minutes. Bake at 350° for approximately 15 – 20 minutes, or until golden brown. Serve warm.

Tip: For moister rolls, you can brush the rolls with additional honey-butter sauce immediately after they come out of the oven.

Dill Potato Bread

An aromatic, hearty, grounding bread for cooler weather.

Preparation time: 40 minutes
Cooking time: 10–15 minutes
Rising time: 70 minutes
Baking time: 30–40 minutes
Preheat oven to 350°

Makes: 2 loaves
Autumn, Winter

Boil in 3 cups water:

2 medium russet potatoes, peeled and cubed

Discard water, mash potatoes, and let cool to room temperature.

Mix in a small bowl and let foam for 10 minutes:

1½ cups lukewarm water
2 tablespoons active dry yeast
⅛ cup honey

Mix in a large bowl:

mashed potatoes (at most 3 cups)
2 tablespoons honey
¼ cup olive oil
2 teaspoons salt
½ cup green onions, minced
3 cups unbleached white flour
3 cups whole wheat flour
2 tablespoons dried dill weed

Mix all ingredients together to form a dough. Place on floured surface and knead for 10 minutes and let rise for 40 minutes or until doubled in size. Punch down and shape into two round loaves. Place on oiled baking trays, cover, and let rise another 30 minutes. Brush with melted butter or ghee or egg-wash. Using a sharp knife, create three slits in the top of the loaves. Bake at 350° for 30–40 minutes.

Garlic Potato Bread

Thin, light, and crispy—it looks a bit like a pizza crust, and it has a Middle-Eastern flavor. Great with Hummus and green salad.

Preparation time: 40 minutes
Cooking time: 15 minutes
Rising time: 50 minutes
Baking time: 15 – 25 minutes
Preheat oven to 350°

Makes: one 12" round flat bread
Spring, Summer

Boil in water until soft, but not mushy:

1 large russet potato, peeled and cubed

Strain and save water. Let cool to room temperature. Set aside.

In a small bowl, mix and let foam for 10 minutes:

1 cup lukewarm potato water
1 tablespoon active dry yeast
1 teaspoon honey

In a large bowl, combine:

cooked potato, mashed
1 clove garlic, peeled and minced
1 cup whole wheat flour
1½ cups unbleached white flour
1 teaspoon salt

Add active dry yeast mixture to flour mixture and combine thoroughly. Knead for 10 minutes. Put in a well buttered bowl, and brush top with generous amount of soft butter or ghee. Cover and let rise until size is doubled (approximately 30 minutes). Punch down the dough and roll to about ½" thickness (should be round and flat, like a pizza).Place in an oiled 12" round pizza baking pan. Make dimples on surface of dough with fingertips.

Brush the top of the dough with soft butter or ghee again and let rise for about 20 minutes. Before baking, you can sprinkle the top with rosemary. Bake at 350° for 15 – 25 minutes, or until golden brown. It should be light and fluffy.

Sun-Dried Tomato Bread

Hearty treat on a cold day.

Soaking time: 20 minutes
Preparation time: 35 minutes
Rising time: 50 minutes
Baking time: 25 – 30 minutes
Preheat oven to 350°

Makes: 2 round loaves
Autumn, Winter

Boil 3 cups water and pour into a bowl with:

1½ cups sun-dried tomatoes

Soak for 20 minutes.

Drain water and drizzle olive oil over tomatoes to coat.

Mix in a small bowl and let foam for 10 minutes:

2 cups lukewarm water
1 tablespoon active dry yeast
1 teaspoon honey

Mix in a large bowl:

soaked sun-dried tomatoes, minced
1 cup semolina flour
2 cups whole wheat flour (or whole wheat pastry flour)
4 cups unbleached white flour
1 tablespoon salt

Add foamy yeast mixture to flour bowl and mix until dough is created. Knead for 10 minutes and place in well oiled bowl (remember to turn dough so both top and bottom are oiled). Cover and let rise for 30 minutes or until dough doubles in size. Punch dough down and shape into 2 round loaves (about 1½" high). Place on oiled baking trays, cover, and let rise 20 minutes. Brush with egg-wash and bake at 350° for 25 – 30 minutes.

Yam Cornbread

A hearty, nourishing bread with a golden color that appeals to the eye. Goes well with any of our vegetable soups.

Preparation time: 40 minutes
Cooking time: 10 minutes
Rising time: 1 hour
Baking time: 30 – 35 minutes
Preheat oven to 350°

Makes: 2 large loaves
Autumn, Winter

Boil in 1 cup water until soft:

½ medium yam, peeled and cut into chunks (enough to make 1-cup mashed yam)

Once soft, discard water and mash yam. Set aside to cool.

In a small bowl, combine:

2 tablespoons active dry yeast
1½ cups warm water
1 teaspoon honey

Let foam for 10 minutes. Then add to active dry yeast mixture:

1 cup corn meal
1 cup unbleached white flour

Mix well and let rise for 30 minutes.

In a separate bowl, combine:

2 cups boiling water
2 cups corn meal

Let sit for 5 minutes. In another bowl, mix:

4½ cups unbleached white flour
1½ teaspoons salt
¼ cup sunflower, or olive oil
1 cup mashed yam

Combine the corn meal and water mixture with the yam mixture. Fold in the active dry yeast mixture. Mix well, place on floured surface then knead for 10 minutes. Let rise for

30 minutes (or until doubled in size) and punch down.

Cut dough in half and shape each half into a round loaf. Place on oiled baking tray, cover, and let rise 30 minutes in a warm place. Brush top with melted butter or ghee, and sprinkle with sesame seeds. Bake at 350° for 30–35 minutes.

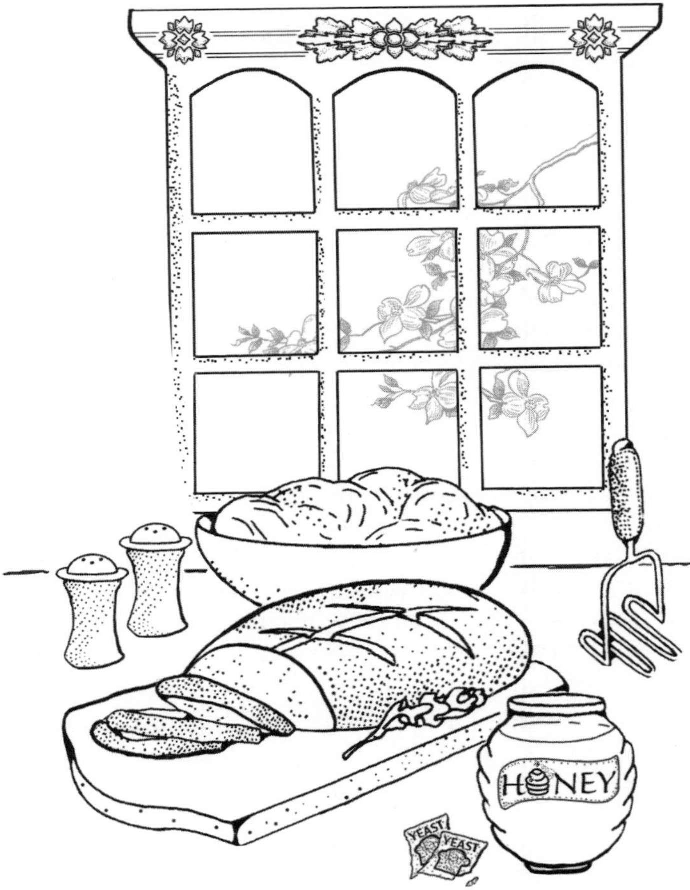

Focaccia

A leavened, flat, Italian bread—light and crisp.

Preparation time: 25 minutes
Rising time: 60 – 90 minutes
Baking time: 20 minutes
Preheat oven to 425°

Makes: One 12″ x 18″ baking tray or 24 triangular pieces
All Year

Place in a bowl, stir and then let stand for 5 – 10 minutes:

3 cups lukewarm water
2 tablespoons active dry yeast
2 teaspoons honey

When mixture becomes foamy add:

¼ cup olive oil

Mix in a large bowl:

3 cups whole wheat flour
4 cups unbleached white flour
2 teaspoons salt
1 tablespoon fresh rosemary, minced, or 1 teaspoon dried rosemary (optional)

Add yeast mixture to dry ingredients and mix well. Knead for 5 minutes by hand. Place dough in an oiled bowl, turn dough to coat with oil. Cover with plastic wrap and let rise for 40 – 60 minutes or until doubled in size. Turn dough out onto oiled baking tray (12" by 18"). With flattened hand, spread dough gently out from center to the edges. Make sure dough is fairly level. Make dimples on surface of dough with finger tips. Drizzle or brush approximately 2 tablespoons olive oil over top.

Let rise a second time for approximately 20 minutes. Then bake at 425° for 20 minutes or until dough sounds hollow when tapped. Remove from tray and cool on rack.

Serving idea: Cut into 24 triangular pieces. To do this make 2 lengthwise cuts and then 3 crosswise cuts to create 12 pieces. Then cut each piece diagonally in half.

Variations:

1. For herbed focaccia add to dry ingredients:

2 teaspoons dried oregano
2 teaspoons dried marjoram
2 teaspoons dried basil.

2. Before the second rising, place sliced tomatoes (or cherry tomatoes cut in half—red or yellow), on surface of dough and gently press into dough. For cherry tomatoes, place the cut side down. Let rise, sprinkle with salt and bake.

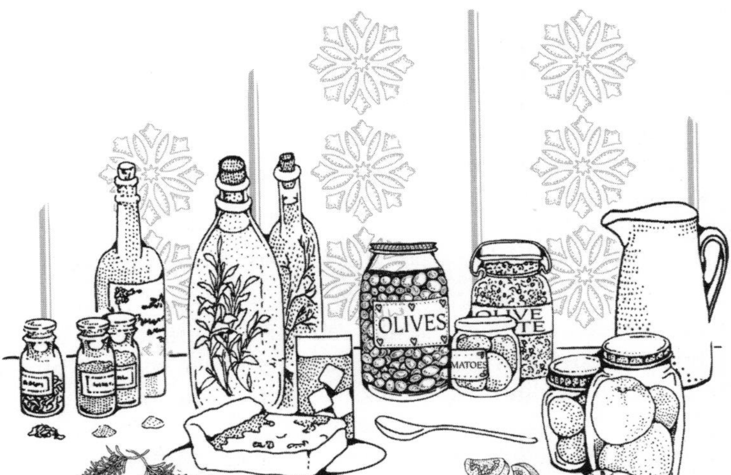

Rye Bread & Rolls

Slightly sweet flavor, very tasty. Goes well with soups, particularly Squash Soup.

Preparation time: 30 minutes
Rising time: 90 minutes

Makes: 2 loaves
or 18 rolls
Spring, Autumn, Winter

Baking time: 15 minutes for rolls; 30 – 35 minutes for loaves
Preheat oven to 350°

Mix:

2 cups water
1 tablespoon active dry yeast
1 tablespoon honey or molasses

Let foam for 10 minutes.

Add:

1 large orange (juice and rind)*
3 tablespoons honey or molasses
2 tablespoons sunflower oil
1½ cups whole wheat flour
4 cups unbleached white flour
2½ cups rye flour
1 teaspoon salt
1½ tablespoons anise seeds (or 2 teaspoons fennel seeds and 3 teaspoons caraway seeds)

Mix the ingredients, place on floured surface and knead for 10 minutes. Cover with a damp towel and let rise for 60 minutes or until doubled in size. Punch down and shape into either 2 round loaves (place on oiled baking trays) or 18 rolls (shape into balls and place in oiled muffin tins in cloverleaf pattern—see Appendix B, page 186). For a variation, this bread can also be shaped in a knot or a figure "8" (see Appendix B. page 183). Let rise again for 30 minutes. Brush with egg-wash and sprinkle with poppy seeds (optional).

Bake at 350° for 15 minutes for rolls and 30–35 minutes for loaves.

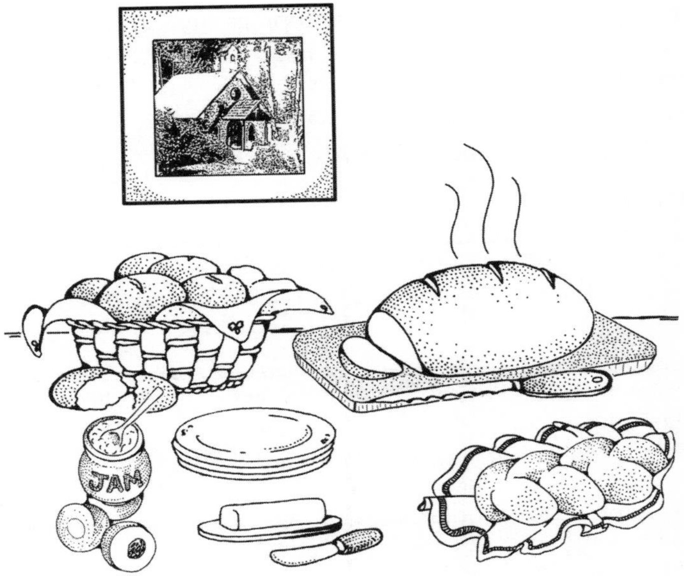

**Juice and rind of orange: First wash and peel off the outermost skin (rind) and finely chop it; then cut orange in half and squeeze the juice.*

Suggested Menus

The menus below were formed around the recipes in this cookbook. Each menu combines grain, protein, and/or vegetables whose colors, textures, and tastes complement one another. We offer 2–4 dish menus for all occasions. Some of the menus include a simple dish such as a steamed vegetable, even though recipes are not given in the book for these suggestions. Note: in the list below, the titles of recipes in this book are capitalized, those not in this book are italicized.

For a balanced, healthy diet, it's good to have both cooked and raw foods. At *The Expanding Light* we always offer with lunch and dinner a fresh, raw green salad: romaine lettuce and assorted greens with toppings such as cucumbers, tomatoes, carrots, jicama, sprouts, and a variety of salad dressings. Use your own favorite raw salads with the menus below.

Spring and Summer

Lunches

Tofu Spinach Pie Cilantro Beets	Barley Salad Sweet Basil Carrots
Mexican Vegetables Mexican Rice or Poppyseed Cornbread	Pasta with Tomato Pizza Sauce Walnut Balls
Bulgur Garbanzo Salad Sweet Zucchini Salad or Tomato Basil Salad	

Pinto Beans Italiano Magic Vegetable Topping Plain Rice	Pad Thai Focaccia
Summer Rice Salad Tofu Salad Raw Kale Salad	Potato Leek Salad or Roasted Potatoes Greek Spinach Frittata
Rice with Red Bell Peppers Pesto Vinaigrette Garbanzo “Croutons” Stuffed Mushrooms	Plain Rice with Pasta Pesto Vinaigrette Roasted Eggplant with Tomato
Hummus Garlic Potato Bread Sweet Zucchini Salad	Stuffed Zucchini Cilantro Beets Aduki Bean Salad *corn on the cob*
Spinach Mushroom Sauce Tofu Salad *baked potatoes* *steamed broccoli*	Pesto Pasta Sweet Zucchini Salad Focaccia Radish Romaine Salad
Simple Tasty Plain Rice Baked Zucchini White Bean Spread Sun Dried Tomato Bread Tomato Basil Salad	Rosemary Olive Bread Roasted Eggplant with Balsamic Dressing Garbanzo “Croutons”
Garbanzo Vegetable Curry Plain Rice Cucumber Raita	Millet Patties Mushroom Gravy *steamed bok choy*

Spring and Summer

Dinners

Warm Couscous Salad Seasoned Spinach Salad	Thai Stir Fry Focaccia
Cauliflower Soup Basic Whole Wheat Bread or Whole Wheat Biscuits	Quinoa Salad *artichokes* Herbed Ghee
Potato Garlic Spread Whole Wheat Sesame Crackers Raw Kale Salad or Radish Romaine Salad	Navy White Bean Spread Whole Wheat Sesame Crackers Salad with Orange Shallot Dressing
Potato-Mushroom Soup Sunflower Kale Salad Carrot or Yam Pillows	Corn Bisque Spinach Stuffed Bread or Sesame Rolls
Pizza (use Whole Wheat Bread for crust) Pesto Sauce Tomato Pizza Sauce	Garbanzo Stew Plain Bulgur
Miso Soup Nori Rolls Dipping Sauce	Plain Rice Zucchini-Carrot Sauce Garbanzo "Croutons"

Autumn and Winter

Lunches

Vegetable Empanada Tahini Sauce Plain Quinoa	Vegetable Pasties Tahini Sauce
Veggie Paté Apricot Dijon Sauce or Golden Gravy	Millet Patties Tahini Sauce *steamed broccoli*
Aduki Bean Salad Eggplant Tahini Potato Leek Salad Sweet Zucchini Salad (serve salads warm)	Vegetable Wraps Sweet Tomato Sauce Indian Herbed Rice Date Raisin Chutney
Butternut Coconut Soup Lemon Rice Maple Sesame Tofu	Barley Salad Savory Tofu Cilantro Beets
Cauliflower Millet Tahini Sauce Dill Butternut Squash Sunflower Kale Salad	Stuffed Cabbage Sweet Tomato Sauce or Lemon Tomato Sauce Cilantro Beets
Simple Tasty Rice Herbed Vegetables Hummus	Colorful Baked Vegetables Hummus Plain Rice or Focaccia

Rice Patties Mushroom Gravy Dill Butternut Squash Savory Tofu	Lentil Chile Dhal Vegetables in Coconut Curry Sauce Plain Rice Cucumber Raita *whole wheat chappatis*
Vegetable Tofu Patties Mushroom Gravy Gingered Yams	Tofu Puff Pasties Mushroom Gravy Carrot Pillows Lemon Rice Sweet Zucchini Salad (Exquisite holiday meal)
Yam Delight Aduki Bean Salad Lemon Rice	Baked Fennel Bulbs Cilantro Beets Garbanzo Croutons or Navy Bean Spread Festive Rice
Moroccan Stew Cucumber Raita Plain Rice or Plain Bulgur	

Autumn and Winter

Dinners

Udon Vegetable Soup Dill Potato Bread	Spinach Yam Soup Rye Rolls or Whole Wheat Bread
Barley Vegetable Soup Whole Wheat Biscuits	Barley Salad Burdock Root and Carrots
Split Pea Soup Cilantro Beets or Gingered Yams Seasoned Spinach Salad Plain Rice	Red Lentil Soup Barley Bread Sauteéd Turnips or Seasoned Spinach Salad
Green Bean Soup Whole Wheat Bread or Dill Potato Bread Tofu Salad	Garbanzo Soup Sesame Sticks *steamed broccoli or kale*
Kitchari Apple Chutney	Squash Soup Dill Potato Bread Savory Tofu
Red Lentil Soup Whole Wheat Bread or Indian Herbed Rice Sunflower Kale Salad	

Appendix A
Vegetable Cutting Shapes

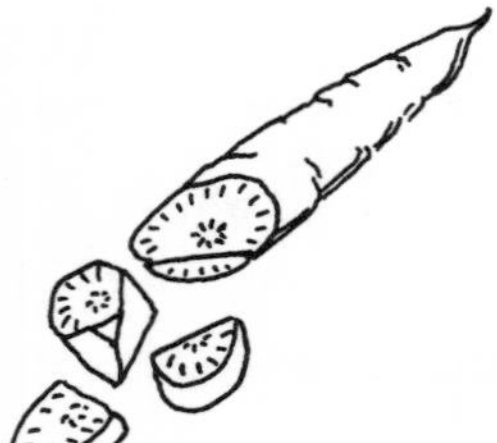

Chunks

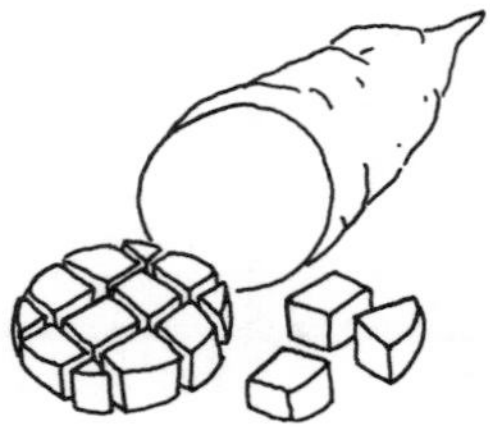

Cubes

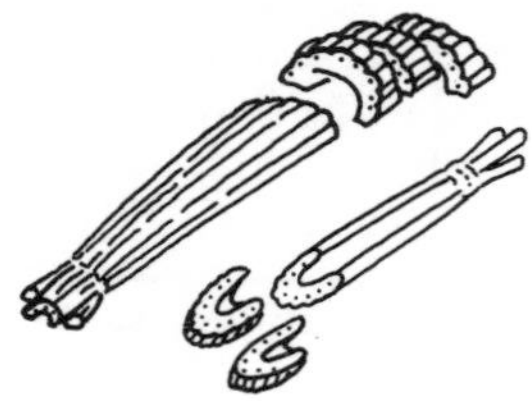

Diagonals

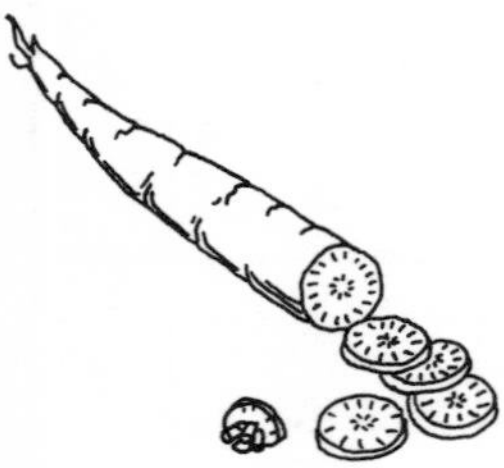

Rounds

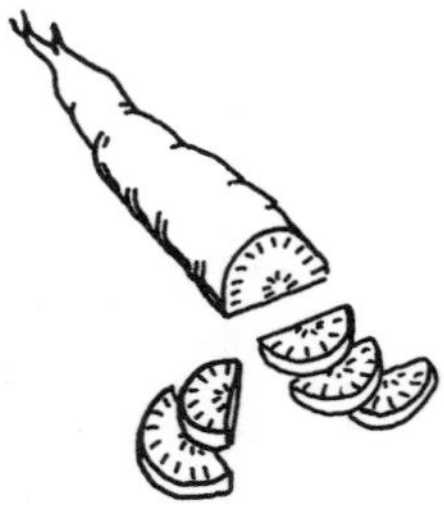

Half Rounds

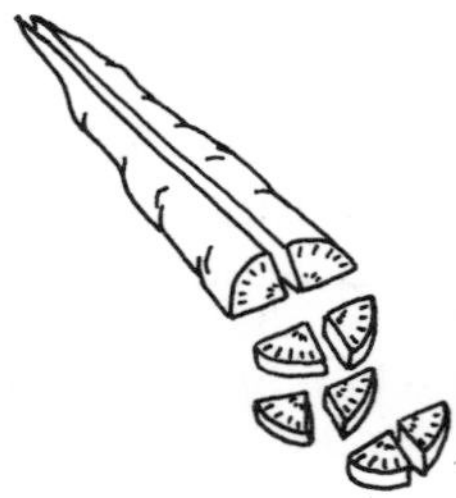

Quarter Rounds

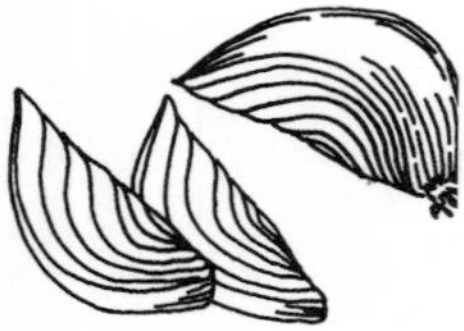

Crescents

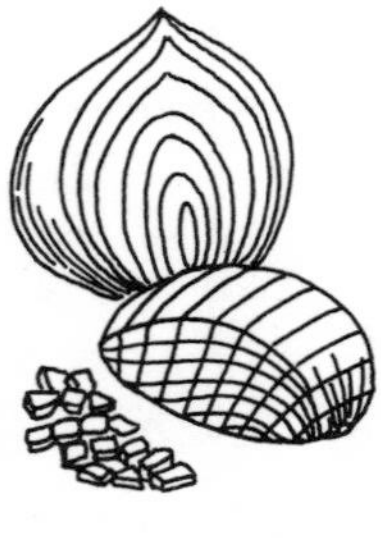

Minced

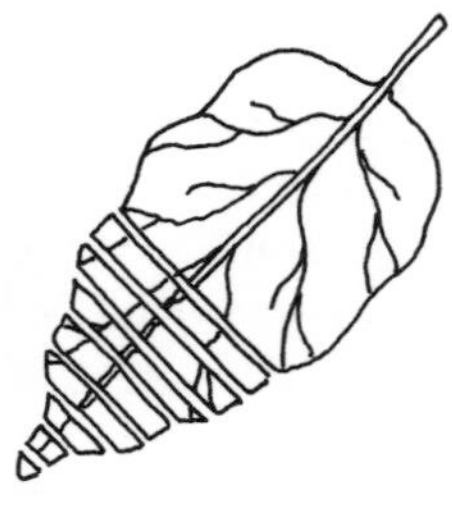

Strips

Appendix B
Shapes for Breads and Rolls

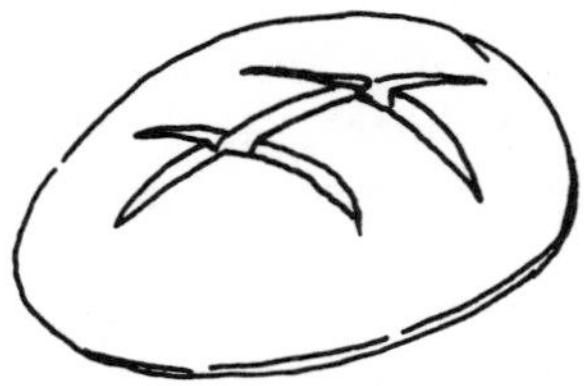

Round Loaf

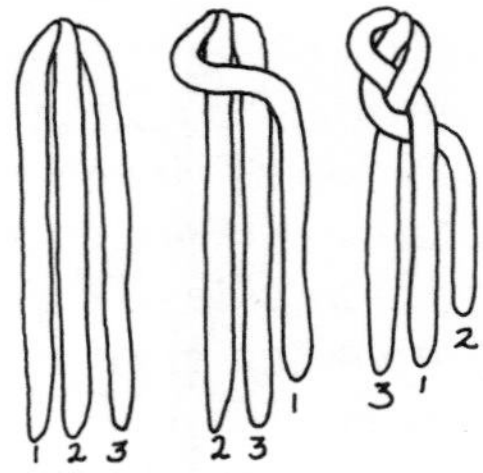

Braided Bread

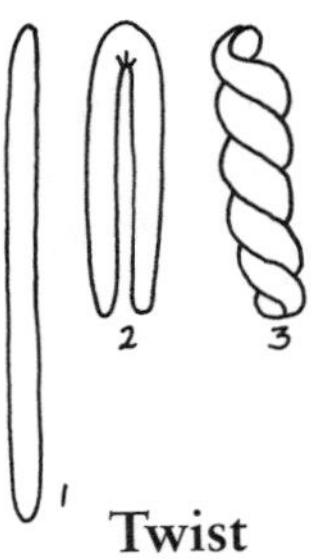

Twist

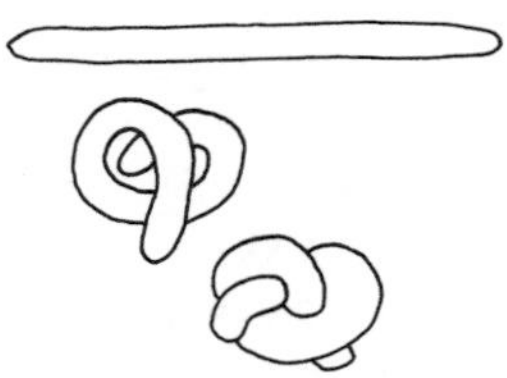

Knot

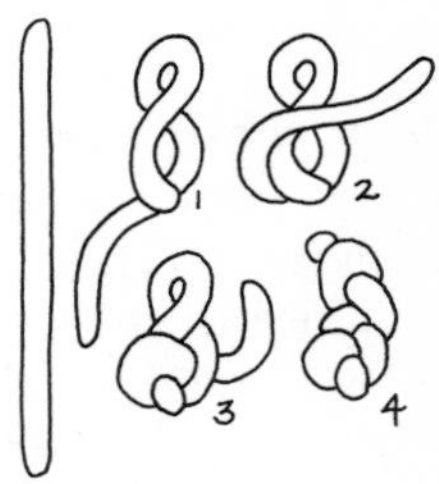

Figure "8"

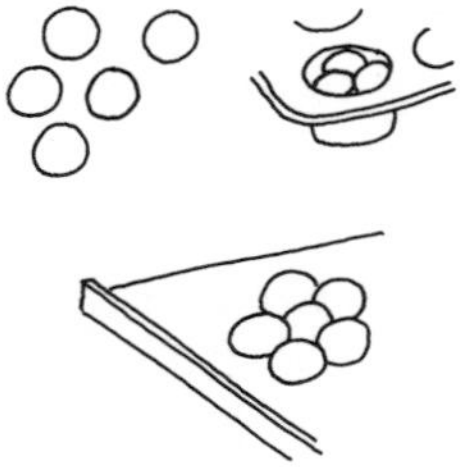

Cloverleaf Balls

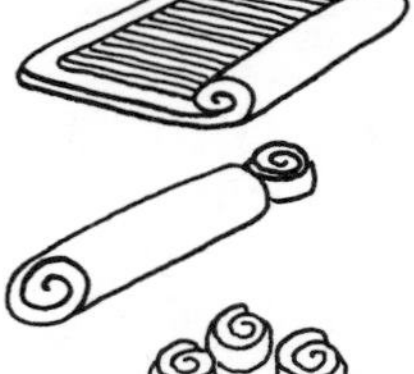

Cinnamon Rolls

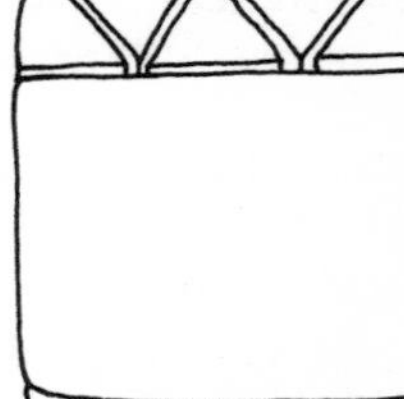

Pillows

Appendix C

How to Make Ghee

Ghee is an ideal cooking oil, as it does not burn unless heated excessively. It is used instead of butter and keeps without refrigeration. People who are allergic to dairy products are unable to enjoy butter, but some can tolerate ghee. Commercial ghee is available at health food stores and Indian groceries, but it's easy and more economical to make your own.

Cooking time: 40 – 50 minutes All Year

Place in a heavy sauce pan (preferably stainless steel):
1 pound (or 4 sticks) unsalted butter—regular or raw

Melt the butter and cook over medium to low heat (best to use a flame diffuser if possible) so that the butter just boils gently. (Do not cover the pot.) A foam of milk solids will rise to the surface; do not skim off or stir. After about 30 – 40 minutes, the foam will settle to the bottom of the pot, where it will create a thick layer. At this point, watch the ghee carefully to avoid burning. When the bottom layer turns a light tan color and the liquid becomes clear and golden, the ghee has formed. With a flame diffuser, the whole process takes 40–50 minutes. Remove from heat and let cool. Pour the contents of the pot through a fine sieve into a glass container for storage.

Note: After ghee is done and has cooled, keep it covered and avoid using a wet spoon, or allowing any water to mix with it, as that will create the conditions for bacteria to grow and spoil the ghee. Burnt ghee has a nutty smell and a brownish color; it can still be used if not burned excessively.

Appendix D

How to Make Patties

Patties are a familiar yet creative way to eat grains and tofu—see recipes in the "Beans & Tofu" and "Grains" sections.

Since our patties do not include eggs, it is important to make sure that the mixture is wet and sticky. If needed, add a little water or vegetable broth and/or oil.

We have found that using a jam jar ring is easier, faster, and more uniform when shaping the patties. For measuring quantities, a 3½" diameter ring is a good size to use. Scoop some of the mixture with a spoon, and press firmly into the ring to create a patty. Distribute patties ½" apart on oiled baking tray. Bake at 350° in the middle of the oven for about 20 minutes until golden. Patties are good with your favorite gravy. (Serve 2 patties per person as a main dish).

If you do not have a jam jar ring, shape patties by scooping the mixture with a big spoon onto an oiled tray. Baking the patties is a healthy alternative to deep frying. Baking also saves time and does not compromise taste.

Appendix E

Glossary

Arrowroot powder: A natural thickening agent.

Bragg Liquid Aminos: A liquid vegetable protein made from pure soybeans and purified water. Flavoring similar to tamari with a low sodium content—unfermented, a good source of amino acids.

Bulgur: Whole wheat that has been steamed, dried, and cracked.

Burdock root: This carrot like root vegetable is brown-skinned with white flesh. It is always served cooked and has an earthy aroma and flavor. Medicinally it is said to be a blood purifier and strengthening to the kidneys. Can be found in Asian grocery stores and some health food stores.

Couscous: A refined grain made from the endosperm remnants of refined durum wheat. Whole wheat couscous is darker in color than traditional couscous; it is a whole, more nutritious food that is available through natural food stores and some supermarkets.

Fennel: A member of the parsley family. Has a round, pale green bulb, short stems, and feathery green leaves. Has a mild, sweet flavor akin to licorice or anise. Because of its taste, fennel is called "anise" in many markets, but it is an entirely different plant from the herb anise. Fennel seeds, like the vegetable they come from, have a mild licorice flavor (much milder than anise).

Flame diffuser: A flat metal disk with holes and handle. Placing it between a pan and gas stove burner spreads heat evenly and keeps food from burning or sticking to the bottom of the pan.

Garbanzo beans: Also known as chickpeas.

Ghee: Clarified butter, i.e., butter without the milk solids. Appendix C, page 184, has instructions for making ghee.

Kale: A green leafy vegetable with curly leaves and coarse texture; one of the more nutritious cooking greens. Our recipes specify green kale; other kinds of kale are yellow-green, red, or purple.

Miso: A thick paste made from fermented soybeans and usually a grain such as rice or barley. There are several varieties of miso, which vary in saltiness and strength; our recipes specify "mellow" miso, which is light and not too salty, with a slightly sweet flavor.

Semolina flour: A high-protein flour made from durum wheat.

Spike®: Brand name of a vegetable seasoning.

Tahini: A paste made from hulled sesame seeds. It is sold raw or toasted; our recipes specify raw tahini.

Tamari: A salty liquid (a by-product of soy bean miso) fermented, somewhat like soy sauce. Appropriate for use in cooking.

Tofu: A curd made from soybeans. Our recipes specify "firm" tofu.

Whole Wheat Udon: Wheat noodle from Japan. Available in Asian markets and some natural food stores. Brown rice udon is made from brown rice and wheat.

Index to Recipes

About the Author

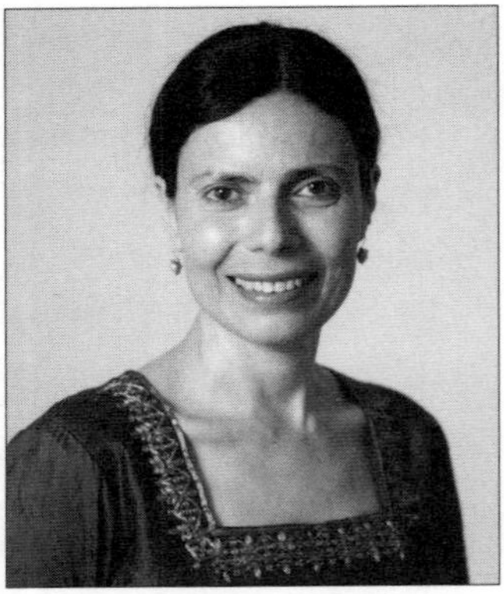

Diksha McCord was the head chef at The Expanding Light Retreat, where she is currently part of the teaching staff. She teaches yoga, meditation, and health classes. She learned vegetarian Kosher cooking while growing up in Israel, studied Temple cooking with Buddhist monks while living in Kyoto, Japan, and learned Ayurvedic, macrobiotic and Indian cooking from premier Californian chefs. Diksha is also the author of the best-selling title *Vegetarian Cooking for Starters*, an excellent resourse containing advice and guidelines for the new vegetarian as well as delicious low-fat recipes.

She lives in Northern California with her husband, Gyandev Rich McCord.

About The Expanding Light

Visited by over two thousand people each year, The Expanding Light welcomes seekers from all backgrounds. Here you will find a loving, accepting environment, ideal for personal growth and spiritual renewal. We offer a varied, year-round schedule of classes and workshops. Offerings include: yoga, meditation, spiritual practices, yoga and meditation teacher training, and personal renewal retreats.

We strive to create an ideal relaxing and supportive environment for people to explore their own spiritual growth. We share the nonsectarian meditation practices and yoga philosophy of Paramhansa Yogananda and his direct disciple, Ananda's founder, Swami Kriyananda. Yogananda called his path "Self-realization," and our goal is to help our guests tune in to their own higher Self. Guests at The Expanding Light can learn the four practices that comprise Yogananda's teachings of Kriya Yoga: the Energization Exercises, the Hong Sau technique of concentration, the AUM technique, and Kriya Yoga. The first two techniques are available for all guests; the second two are available to those interested in pursuing this path more deeply.

Contact Information:

mail: 14618 Tyler Foote Rd., Nevada City, CA 95959

phone: 800-346-5350

online: www.expandinglight.org

email: info@expandinglight.org

Further Resources

Crystal Clarity Publishers Books

Vegetarian Cooking for Starters

Blanche Agassy McCord (Diksha McCord)

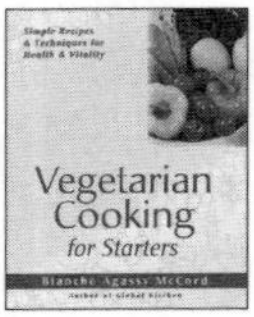

Are you confused by the many different foods, theories, fads, and techniques championed by various proponents of healthy eating? In *Vegetarian Cooking for Starters*, McCord gives straightforward, easy-to-follow dietary advice, explains what common vegetarian foods are, offers immediately useful explanations on how to prepare vegetarian dishes, and includes simple, savory recipes that will quickly help you add vegetarian meals to your diet.

Autobiography of a Yogi

Paramhansa Yogananda

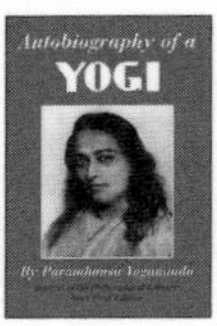

Autobiography of a Yogi—one of the best-selling Eastern philosophy titles of all time, with millions of copies sold—was named one of the best and most influential books of the twentieth century. This highly prized reprinting of the original 1946 edition is the only one available free from textual changes made after Yogananda's death.Yogananda was the first yoga master of India whose mission was to live and teach in the West. His account of his life experiences includes childhood revelations, stories of his visits to saints and masters in India, and long-secret teachings of Self-realization that he made available to the reader.

Living Wisely Living Well

Swami Kriyananda

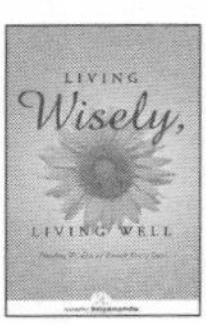

Learn the art of spiritual living. Do you want to transform your life? Tap your highest potential? Get inspired, uplifted, and motivated? *Living Wisely, Living Well* contains 366 practical ways to improve your life—a thought for each day of the year. Each saying is war with wisdom, alive with positive expectation, and provides simple actions that bring profound results. See life with new eyes. Discover hundreds of techniques for self-improvement. Take a year off from the "same old you." Read this book, put into practice what it teaches, and in a year's time you won't recognize yourself.

Meditation for Starters

Swami Kriyananda

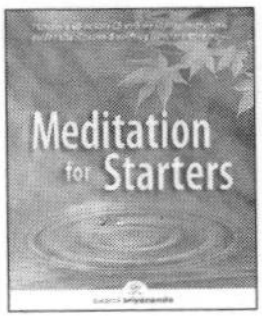

Have you wanted to learn to meditate, but just never got around to it? Or tried "sitting in the silence" only to find yourself too restless to stay more than a few moments? If so, *Meditation for Starters* is just what you've been looking for—and with a companion CD, it provides everything you need to begin a meditation practice. It is filled with easy-to-follow instructions, beautiful guided visualizations, and answers to important questions on meditation, such as what meditation is (and isn't); how to relax your body and prepare yourself for going within; and techniques for interiorizing and focusing the mind.

Affirmations for Self-Healing

Swami Kriyananda

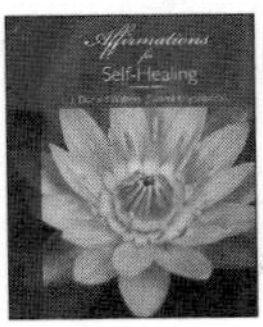

This inspirational book contains fifty-two affirmations and prayers, each pair devoted to improving a quality in ourselves. Strengthen your will power; cultivate forgiveness, patience, health, and enthusiasm. A powerful tool for self-transformation.

Music Selections

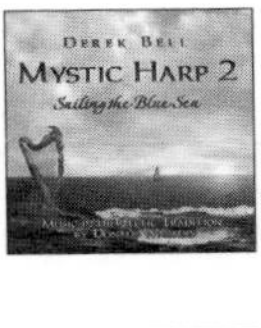

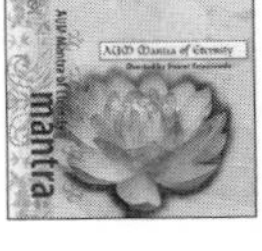

The Mystic Harp 1 & 2—Derek Bell

Derek Bell, of Ireland's five-time Grammy Award winning **Chieftains**, captures the haunting, mystical quality of traditional Celtic music on this solo album of original melodies by Donald Walters (Swami Kriyananda). Derek plays Celtic harp on each richly orchestrated melodies on both albums.

AUM: Mantra of Eternity—Swami Kriyananda

Mantra of Eternity features continuous vocal chanting of "Aum," set to tamboura accompaniment. Aum (pronounced OM) is the sound that emanates from the heart of creation, bringing consciousness into outer manifestation, maintaining it, and dissolving it back again, finally, into Infinite Spirit. By attuning one's consciousness to this sound, one enters the stream of vibration that proceeded out of Spirit and that merges back into Spirit at creation's end.

Crystal Clarity Publishers

When you're seeking a book on practical spiritual living, you want to know it's based on an authentic tradition of timeless teachings, and that it resonates with integrity. This is our goal: to offer you books of practical wisdom filled with true spiritual principles that have not only been tested through the ages, but also through personal experience. We only publish books that combine creative thinking, universal principles, and a timeless message. Crystal Clarity books will open doors to help you discover more fulfillment and joy by living and acting from the center of peace within you.

Crystal Clarity Publishers—recognized worldwide for its bestselling, original, unaltered edition of Paramhansa Yogananda's classic *Autobiography of a Yogi*—offers many additional resources to assist you in your spiritual journey, including over one hundred books and a wide variety of inspirational and relaxation music composed by Swami Kriyananda, Yogananda's direct disciple, and yoga and meditation DVDs.

In addition to our music and audiobook offerings, many of our book titles are available in unabridged MP3 format audiobooks and can be downloaded on our full-service secure website. Or, look for us in the popular online download sites.

To request a catalog, place an order for the products you read about in the Further Resourcess section of this book, or to obtain more information about us and our products, please contact us:

Contact Information:

mail: 14618 Tyler Foote Rd., Nevada City, CA 95959

phone: 800-424-1055 or 530-478-7600

online: www.crystalclarity.com

email: clarity@crystalclarity.com

Ananda Sangha Worldwide

A worldwide fellowship of kindred souls following the teachings of Paramhansa Yogananda, the Sangha embraces the search for higher consciousness through the practice of meditation, and through the ideal of service to others in their quest for Self-realization. Approximately ten thousand spiritual seekers are affiliated with Ananda Sangha throughout the world.

Founded in 1968 by Swami Kriyananda, a direct disciple of Paramhansa Yogananda, Ananda includes seven communities in the United States, Europe, and in India. Worldwide, about one thousand devotees live in these spiritual communities, which are based on Yogananda's ideals of "plain living and high thinking."

Swami Kriyananda lived with his guru during the last four years of the Master's life, and continued to serve his organization for another ten years, bringing the teachings of Kriya Yoga and Self-realization to audiences in the United States, Europe, Australia, and, from 1958–1962, India. In 1968, together with a small group of close friends and students, he founded the first "world brotherhood community" in the foothills of the Sierra Nevada Mountains in Northern California.

After more then forty years of existence, Ananda is one of the most successful networks of intentional communities in the world. Urban communities have been developed in Palo Alto and Sacramento, California; Portland, Oregon; and Seattle, Washington. In Europe, near Assisi, Italy, nearly one hundred residents from eight countries live. In India, work has begun to develop both urban and rural communities, a retreat center, schools, and a temple dedicated to Paramhansa Yogananda. Ananda Sangha also supports more than one hundred meditation groups worldwide.

Contact Information:

mail: 14618 Tyler Foote Rd., Nevada City, CA 95959

phone: 530-478-7560

online: www.ananda.org

email: sanghainfo@ananda.org